POLAR EXTREMES

*From the Darkness of Bipolar
Disorder to Daylight*

Steve West

To Rob —
all my best,
Steve West

Polar Extremes: From the Darkness of Bipolar Disorder to Daylight
Copyright © 2018 by Stephen G. West.

Cover designed by Chris Harrington

The author has tried to recreate events and timelines with complete accuracy based on official hospital records, a personal journal, related work documents, his own recollections, and those of other sources familiar with this true account. In order to maintain the anonymity and privacy of others, he has changed the names of all individuals and places. Because this story involves a mental illness, the author attempts to differentiate between reality and hallucinations throughout the course of the book for credibility sake wherever possible.

Steve West

Library of Congress by Stephen Gerard West. Catalog Number pending.
Printed in the United States of America

First Printing: January 2019

ISBN 9781798763032

In loving memory of my brothers, Bobby and John; my father, Robert; and my mother, Lucia. To my remaining six siblings and seventeen nieces and nephews. And to the football legend, Archie Manning, who served as my childhood role model both on and off the field.

FOREWORD

When my younger brother, Steve, asked me to write the foreword to his book, I hesitated. Not because of the time it would take, but rather because I didn't like to revisit our childhood, which has profoundly affected us. I preferred not to go down that rabbit hole. I escaped from it years ago, but there is always the fear that once you return to that abyss, you may never have the strength to recover.

Much has been said regarding the impact of heredity and environment on a developing child. You'd have to experience it to understand the day-to-day influence on a child's psyche when trapped in surroundings in which a violent father with a mental disorder locks horns with a mother with a provocative nature. This was surely an unstable situation for eight helpless children who were exposed to a lot of ups and downs . . . an abundance of highs and lows. It created the perfect setting for the development of the disorder of highs and lows, bipolar.

All eight of us suffered repercussions from our upbringing. Each developed our own coping mechanisms to deal with the turmoil. Most of us survived; one did not, but each of us has carried our share of pain.

When you first see a loved one in an active bipolar episode, it is very difficult to process and understand. During my brother's final episode, there were times that I did not know if he'd survive. I'd call the facility where he was housed every other day and I was told he was in a "backroom." They wouldn't say much other than he was unresponsive to the treatment. Five or six weeks passed before I could see him. I remember picking him up and seeing him in such a depleted state. It was heartbreaking.

Thankfully, he has stayed on his medications and has reached out to family members when he doesn't feel right. This is important, because deep in my heart, I know he will not survive another major episode. I am optimistic now that he has been able to write and share his story. I hope it heals some of his wounds, and it helps others struggling with the disorder.

As much as I understand the reasons that my brother wound up at this place, I remain angry that my parents had no regard for how their actions affected my siblings and me. But they say that through pain comes growth, and I am grateful for that which I have witnessed in my brother. I hope you obtain some insight into the disorder by reading the following pages.

Mary Bawarski

PREFACE

T his book includes sixteen "Clinical Overviews" that will offer important medical insight to the reader concerning bipolar disorder. There is one researched topic at the end of each chapter. These educational sections, involving such areas as suicidal and homicidal ideation, will help to remove the mystery and stigma surrounding mental illness. They are as follows:

Chapter one: What are the definitions and symptoms of bipolar disorder?

Chapter two: What is suicidal ideation and its effect on bipolar disorder?

Chapter three: Is there a link between early childhood trauma and bipolar disorder? Is the diagnosis of bipolar disorder different in children and adults?

Chapter four: Is there a link between alcohol/drug abuse and the treatment of bipolar disorder?

Chapter five: What are some of the risks associated with discontinuing bipolar medication?

Chapter six: What are the effects of religious/spiritual beliefs on the treatment of bipolar disorder and other mental illnesses?

Chapter seven: What is homicidal ideation and its link to bipolar disorder and other mental illnesses?

Chapter eight: Is there a correlation between musical and artistic creativity and bipolar disorder?

Chapter nine: Where can you locate information to help educate your friends and the public about bipolar disorder?

Chapter ten: How can a caregiver assist a patient who has experienced a change in lifestyle or job loss because of bipolar disorder?

Chapter eleven: How can a person diagnosed with bipolar disorder best cope with this mental illness?

Chapter twelve: Why is it critical to educate the police concerning the signs of mental illnesses such as bipolar disorder?

Chapter thirteen: What are the similarities and differences between bipolar disorder and schizophrenia?

Chapter fourteen: Is Electroconvulsive Therapy (ECT) a safe alternative for treating bipolar disorder?

Chapter fifteen: What is Parkinson's disease and its link to bipolar disorder?

Chapter sixteen: What are the health risks involved with misdiagnosis of bipolar disorder? Should there be liabilities for doctors who prescribe wrong medications?

Table of Contents

FIRST EPISODE

CHAPTER ONE FIRST EPISODE – PART 1 SEPTEMBER 1996

I almost lost my balance as I slid down the banister to the third-floor landing of our apartment building.

"Hey look, Becky! I can fly!"

Becky, my across-the-hall neighbor, was frantically dialing the phone and casting worried glances in my direction. It was a weekday morning, and she had been sipping tea in her bathrobe before preparing for work when the madness erupted around seven o'clock. And, unfortunately, I was the culprit behind the bizarre chain of events. I was thirty-nine years old at the time.

***

Three years before, I was an eight-year veteran in the salesforce of a major communications company. As a corporate account manager, I was marginal at best, barely attaining my quota each year. But even a blind dog finds a bone now and then. And one day, it was my turn to shine in the sun. My team won a telephone system sale in excess of thirty-two million dollars. It was one of the largest sales in the history of the corporation's New Jersey division.

I learned a thing or two about professional jealousy that day as all my so-called buddies abandoned me one by one. I guess my newfound success precluded me from being part of their clique.

The major sale was for a ten-year contract encompassing thirty-two thousand telephone lines to be installed in thirty-two remote offices and interconnected with sixty-four high speed circuits. This included disaster recovery capabilities.

The customer was a fledgling company that indirectly competed against my corporation for voice communication traffic within the local markets of New Jersey. However, this reseller arrangement allowed us to hold onto a sizeable amount of revenue. These were dollars that we would have otherwise lost to local competitors, such as long-distance carriers. Because of the sale, my client grew significantly. I had essentially put them into business.

A year later, I was demoted from our large to small segment line of business, despite my success, due to political reasons. As a result, I quickly became dissatisfied and decided to look elsewhere for employment. In 1995, Len, the president of the reseller start-up company, offered me a position as sales manager with a substantial raise, which I accepted.

We had a monumental year with record sales and installations, and our business relationship was a huge success. And then it happened.

One day in late 1996, after a significant number of installations had gone smoothly, Len called me into his office and told me to close the door and have a seat.

"Steve, I've decided I'm moving the company in a new direction," he announced, as he removed his glasses and stared straight into my eyes. "Right now, I'm paying you one hundred thousand dollars a year, but the business has stabilized. I can't justify continuing to pay your high salary when I can get someone else in here for half the price."

I was caught totally off guard and momentarily sputtered and squirmed in my chair as I struggled to get the words out.

"But, Len," I said, "I'm the one who put you guys in business in the first place! Isn't there such a thing as loyalty?"

"I'm aware of that," he said, "which is why I'll pay you until you find a new job. I'll have Mitchell get your belongings."

Apparently, he had already given his son the green light because, within seconds, there was a knock on the door. Mitchell tossed a tattered box of my belongings onto the floor. I can still see how my reading glasses were bent, practically in two.

"What about my paintings?" I asked, as if I cared.

"You can come back for those when you pick up your next paycheck," Len said.

There would be no "next paycheck" as he later reneged on his promise.

My mind was in turmoil as I stumbled toward the hallway.

"Oh, and by the way," he said after Mitchell had left the room, "I also didn't like the way you were always giving all the good sales leads to your friend, Jerry. The other sales reps were starting to complain. I wouldn't have minded it if he had closed any of them."

In my opinion, Jerry was our most professional sales rep, which explained my rationale. As the sales manager, I had felt it was my responsibility to the company to generate as much revenue as possible. But now, a white-collared vagabond, I was out on the street. For the first time in my life I had been fired.

As soon as I got to a phone, I called Jerry and told him the news. He had been out in the field that morning and was unaware what had transpired. We agreed to meet at the mall to commiserate.

"It doesn't surprise me, Westy. Len's a sleazebag. You know that. It was bound to happen sooner or later. I may be out of work soon too for all I know."

"It isn't fair."

"You have to calm down; there are other jobs out there. You need to move on. Can I buy you a cup of joe?"

"No. How can you even think about coffee at a time like this? I put the guy in business for crying out loud."

"I'm telling you. Len will get his. Don't make yourself sick over it."

Well, I did make myself sick. Very sick. In fact, Len had managed to almost single-handedly trigger my first episode into the dark, eerie realm of mental illness known as bipolar disorder.

My world literally collapsed overnight. The next morning, I awoke from an agitated sleep in my suburban New Jersey apartment. As I moved in the darkness from my bedroom to living room, I felt the sensation of a rubber band snapping inside my head. The lights seemed to turn themselves on. My perception transformed from black and white into full color, as if I were Dorothy in *The Wizard of Oz*.

My world would never be the same.

I lay down on my bachelor-brown sofa and gazed around the room. My bronze Buddha statue was perched on the radiator ledge. My black Aztec calendar hung on one of the walls. There were four paintings of mine: one portraying *The Beatles in Sergeant Pepper Land*, one of *The Devil's Coven*, a copy of Picasso's *La Guernica,* and one containing symbols, which included the yin and yang. There were multiple framed Egyptian parchments of snakes. The shelves supported statues of the Loch Ness Monster, along with several leprechauns, a gnome and a hairy troll.

Lying there in the still of the early morning it dawned on me for the first time . . . my living room was a veritable museum of the Devil!

My chaotic thoughts had become voices in my head. They would inexplicably return sporadically throughout my current episode. Imagine listening to a radio that was tuned between stations on the dial. They were clear enough that I could pinpoint the source, but the reception was weak and distorted with myriad background noises. I recognized the static in my ears. It was Sonya's voice, an attractive blond former coworker of mine. I had a crush on her.

I could barely discern her faraway words as the source. She was having a conversation with others on the line. Her words weren't directed specifically at me. It was as if I was just listening in.

I covered my ears with both hands to make the torment stop. It only worsened. A second distant voice appeared in the conversation that I recognized. Cliff was also a previous colleague. He had prematurely gray hair and an eccentric personality. As the conspiracy theorist in the company, he was more paranoid then than I was, even now. The intolerable humming was haunting me like the buzzing of a bees nest in my brain. And they wouldn't go away. They were jumbled with the crowds of other internal imaginary voices that I could not distinguish . . . except Priscilla, one of my prior managers.

Without even taking a shower, I hastily donned some dirty clothes, and jumped behind the wheel of my car. Attempting to escape the mind-bending torture with a change of scenery, I somehow made my way to my mother's house in North Arlington.

She and my brother Tim were home in the dining room finishing breakfast. He was carrying dirty dishes to the kitchen sink nearby.

"What's the matter? Are you okay?" she asked.

I guess something in my unkempt appearance signaled there was a problem. The voices had temporarily vanished, but I became suddenly philosophical as we engaged in deep discussion. My mother and Tim were devout Christians, as I claimed to be myself despite my infatuation with statues such as smiling Buddha back home. Our conversation gradually led to our common ground of spirituality.

The words that I spoke didn't sound like my own.

"It's all about freeing up your mind and letting thoughts just flow," I professed in a sophisticated tone. "It's not wise to judge me based on who you think I am."

"What? . . . Are you crazy? Where did you get that from?" she said in her animated Italian accent as she jumped out of her chair. "The Bible says you need to have the wisdom to judge, with an understanding heart, so you can discern between good and bad. Something strange is going on."

"Steve's talking about Buddhism, and meditation, and the yin and yang," said Tim. "Have you been by his apartment lately? I was there the other day. It's like a shrine to the Devil! No wonder he's channeling these crazy thoughts."

I dropped down on my hands and knees and, for some reason, crawled toward Tim at a snail's pace to where he was sitting in the corner recliner. When I reached him, I extended my finger and poked him in the torso. He remained frozen with a frightened look on his face. His palms were gripping the arms of the cushioned chair as he sat in an upright position motionless.

I lifted myself off the tiled floor and wandered silently to the living room where I sprawled out on the couch. My mother and brother followed me warily. She sat in a loveseat while he sat on the carpeted steps, near the telephone. My mind was spiraling like the funnel of a twister preparing to touch down and destroy every obstacle in its path. My mother was wearing a gold cross pendant around her neck. I suddenly jumped and lurched toward her, yanking the chain from her neck.

"You're crazy!" she screamed in terror as she reached in vain to snatch the chain back from my stronger grasp.

I turned toward Tim, growling like a wolverine. He was dialing the telephone. He yelled to my mother that he was going to call his Christian friend for advice on how to proceed. He might need to perform an exorcism. My mother shouted to call the police. But then my mood suddenly lightened, and I became playful, frolicking with miniature leprechaun souvenirs I had purchased during a recent trip in Ireland. I scattered them throughout the house as my brother hesitantly followed me on our demonic scavenger hunt. He sighted one of them under my mother's bed. When he craned to retrieve it, I snuck up behind him and hollered, "Catch me lucky charms!" I doubled over in laughter. He wasn't amused as he placed the tiny statue in his pocket and shook his head in disgust.

Later that same evening I embarked on my next adventure. I called my sister, Vicki, and asked if I could visit her house to see her two young girls, Nicole and Kelly. I rang her from my mother's house after telling Tim my intentions. He called Vicki to "warn" her in advance about my possible antics based on what had just transpired.

"Why do you want to come by?" Vicki asked.

"Because I have some gifts for them."

When I arrived, she was standing in the doorway with my other sister, Marlene. They were smiling but appeared apprehensive, seemingly attempting to contemplate my next move.

They were soon pleasantly surprised when I harmlessly reached into the pocket of my jeans and produced the presents for Nicole and Kelly: ten one-dollar bills. I hid some of them under the couch, and behind the wall unit. Then I climbed upstairs to the children's bedroom, where they were asleep. I woke them up, and they started giggling as I gave each of them a handful of dollars. Shortly thereafter I left the house and was on my way.

My sisters later drove through the center of town at midnight. Cracking open the window, they tossed the money into the street, figuring it was better to be safe than sorry just in case it was demonic, which, by now, had become a recurring theme.

***

Church services were every Sunday morning and Thursday night in town. At this particular weeknight worship, I sensed something was wrong. Years later I would realize that I was experiencing a bipolar episode, having never had one before today. At the time I was only vaguely familiar with the term. Maybe a nervous breakdown would have been more believable. I was amazed by the mood swings between mania and depression.

Prior to the service, I was standing in the parking lot beside my car, next to my brother, Tim. We typically attended church together along with our younger sister, Linda. Tim watched me guardedly as, without warning, I removed a gold tie clasp, engraved with my three initials. I placed it underneath the windshield wiper on the driver's side. Fortunately, he retrieved it. I continued to discard gold jewelry and items throughout my episodes, in some cases permanently.

During the service, I had temporarily lost all inhibitions. I kept sliding over in the pew and poking fellow churchgoers in the leg or in their side as they tried to ignore my odd behavior. I wasn't thrilled about the teachings of this particular church, even when I was coherent. After worship that night, Linda introduced me to the pastor, and I told him my name was Jack.

When he greeted me, I snarled, "Pal, you don't know Jack."

I was quickly and rudely escorted outside by some of the elders, and, once again, my moods were erratic as I began happily strutting up and down the grounds proclaiming in song:

"Oh when the saints come marching in . . ."

I am the world's biggest New Orleans Saints' fan.

Everyone looked at me as if I were crazy. Initially, Linda thought it was comical, but then the church elders encouraged her to take me to the hospital for treatment. She and Tim, who was also present, drove me there still not fully aware as to the reasons behind my erratic behavior.

I likened this unpleasant one-night stay to a scene from a horror movie. For starters, I discarded an extremely expensive piece of gold jewelry with no rational explanation. I straddled the radiator in my hospital room, and removed one of my 24-carat gold cufflinks from my French-cuff shirt. I nonchalantly dropped it down an opening in the top of the metal heating pipes, never to be seen again. Fortunately, I still retained the matching cufflink. Many years later, I would visit a jeweler who designed a perfect replica of the one I had tossed away that night in the hospital. It has served as a constant reminder of the seriousness of my mental illness.

After a few moments, I spun around to discover there was a doctor and nurse looming in the doorway of my room. They were wearing worrisome expressions on their faces. One carried a needle that could have easily harpooned Moby Dick. It quickly became obvious they were on a mission to sedate me for the purpose of strapping me to the bed. However, their thinly-veiled strategy of convincing me to roll over and expose my naked buttocks wasn't working. I refused to budge. After all, I may have been crazy, but I wasn't insane.

As the surreal scene unfolded, Tim and Linda were in the room hovering over me. Tim frowned. He was mumbling and pointing at me. His lips were moving, but I couldn't discern what he was trying to communicate.

Then Linda took her turn. As she stood over me almost menacingly, I suddenly elected to repeat my silly mantra I had used on Tim the other day. I sprang up in bed with a smile and shouted, "Catch me lucky charms!"

Linda started to grin, which quickly developed into full-blown laughter when she realized my intentions were harmless. They must have been forced to leave me there for the night because they soon disappeared. I was too wired to sleep. The doctor and nurse had mysteriously vanished as well, and I celebrated winning the battle of the dreaded needle.

I gazed mischievously out my bedroom door. There was a gentleman sitting behind a desk in the hallway, engrossed in conversation with a uniformed guard. I tiptoed into the hall, seemingly unnoticed. It occurred to me that I must be invisible. I dropped down on my hands and knees and began to crawl across the tiled floor past the desk. Sure enough, they never even glanced in my direction or paused their conversation. I returned to my feet and gingerly made my way toward the exit.

"Hey! Where the hell do you think you're going?" hollered the guard as he came toward me.

The man behind the desk leaped up and sprinted across the hall, cutting me off before I reached the door. They each grabbed me by an arm and dragged me back into my room where I remained quietly for the duration of the night, surprisingly unrestrained, but under a more watchful pair of eyes.

Linda and Tim returned to the hospital the next morning to rescue me from further captivity. Later that night, I heard strange, high frequency beeps in my apartment, which disrupted my sleep. I recall believing that inside Len's building nearby, the Devil's coven was performing rituals. Yes, those were the actual thoughts running through my head. There was no rhyme nor reason to explain them.

I was also convinced that alien satellite dishes were controlling my brain. Sonya, Cliff, and Priscilla's voices were coming in garbled. I had to do something to block out the signals trying to read my mind. I needed some sort of hat. Being a Saints' fan, I searched in my closet and found the sports jersey of my childhood hero, Archie Manning, along with his wool hat. I donned them with jeans and sneakers, and again headed for safety in my mother's house.

Along the way, I drove by Len's site where the Devil worship was transpiring. I removed my gold chain and cross, a gift from my Italian grandmother when I was twelve years old. I threw it on the grounds of their front property to ward off any evil spirits. When I returned a few days later, it was gone. I had foolishly lost this treasured keepsake forever.

Sometime after midnight, I pulled into my mother's driveway about five miles from my home. Treading lightly through her landscaped backyard, I stared into the autumn sky. The temperature was so pleasant for that time of year, fortunate for me, given what occurred next.

In the darkness, I proceeded to take off my clothes, placing them on a picnic table inside the fenced-in property. Under the stars, and in the serenity of the night, I gazed at the sky. I extended my arms towards the heavens, proclaiming in a loud voice:

"I accept the Lord, Jesus Christ, as my savior."

Then I crawled into some nearby hedges and hid, to see if anyone had heard my shouts. There were no rustlings, surprisingly, not even a dog barking. I stood up and headed toward my car in the driveway, leaving my clothes behind in a pile. My family would find my garments the next morning. I imagined some of them would wonder: could it be I had been raptured?

I experienced a sudden urge to go to the bathroom. The sensible decision would have been to simply urinate in the bushes under the cover of darkness, especially since I was already naked. However, my irrational thought process prompted me to enter my mother's house and relieve myself the conventional way, in her bathroom. I discovered the house key, which I knew was kept in the umbrella stand in the foyer. Once inside, I tiptoed over the creaking floor boards and onto the carpeted hallway. My mother's bedroom was directly across from my destination. Fortunately, she was snoring loudly as I made my way inside and pulled the door silently closed behind me. After comforting my bladder, and flushing against my better judgment, I managed to exit the premises undetected.

Upon eventually reaching my car, it dawned on me again that I was unclad, with only two worldly possessions. They were my car keys, which I had left in the ignition of my car, and a light jacket I had thrown into the backseat, prior to my striptease. I drove back to my apartment building nude, praising God for not being pulled over, especially since I was one of only a few cars on the road.

But now I had other problems. Once I reached my building, with my jacket wrapped around the front of my waist, I had no means of getting inside since I had left my house key in the pocket of my jeans in my mother's backyard. Luckily, my friend Becky was a night owl, and I saw the light on in her place. I buzzed her apartment and prayed for a miracle. Thankfully, she came down and let me in with a quizzical expression etched on her face, but without asking why I was half-naked.

In order to understand her passive reaction, you should know that she and I were best friends for close to two years, having initially met through my sister, Linda, who had previously occupied an apartment on our same floor. It was the first time in my life I could recall having a truly platonic relationship with a woman. Becky and I found each other a bit quirky. She sat up until the wee hours of the morning on a regular basis. I would hear laughter filtering though her door as she watched the Bullwinkle and Rocky the Flying Squirrel cartoons. She ate cereal for dinner, and referred to me as "Steve Three" in order to avoid confusion since she was dating two "Steve's" already. We would often exchange dating stories at a local pub within walking distance of our building and close the place in the days just prior to my bipolar disorder diagnosis. Sometimes we would stop for ice cream along the way. She was a lawyer in New York City, and she felt pity for me when I had recently lost my job.

"I misplaced the key to my apartment," I said. "Can I please stay the night on your living room couch with your cats?"

I would explain everything in the morning, which by now, was only a few hours away. "Not a problem," she responded almost matter-of-factly.

She rummaged through her bedroom dresser drawer and found me a pair of sweat pants from an ex-boyfriend. I thanked her and pulled them on, although they were too big.

It was as if the cats sensed I was in a crazed state of mind because they clawed mercilessly at my head throughout the brief night.

When I awoke, Becky was in her bathrobe boiling water in the kitchen in preparation of getting ready for work. "Would you like a cup of tea?"

"No thank you. I don't drink tea, or coffee for that matter."

She sat down on a chair, looked curiously at me, and asked: "So, what's up, then?"

I tried my best to start a normal conversation, but I was simply unable. I could sense I was beginning to lose it again.

"I just haven't been feeling myself lately, and . . . Can I explain some other time?" I fidgeted. I jumped off the couch and made my way toward the door, forgetting momentarily that I didn't have the key to get into my apartment. As I groggily passed her wall unit, I spotted two long wax candles. She was following me out into the hallway when I suddenly pivoted. I held the candles in the sign of a cross and shoved them against her neck and bared my teeth like a vampire.

"Give those back to me!" she shrieked, snatching them from me.

I scurried into the hall, toward the banister. The oversized sweatpants slid down around my ankles.

"Hey look, Becky! I can fly!"

Ed, the superintendent, soon arrived, chuckled momentarily at my nakedness as I stood on the landing below, but then demanded, "What the hell is going on here?"

"I think he has a brain tumor!" screamed Becky.

Fortunately, Ed allowed me into my apartment where I was able to shower and change into a new set of clothes. At my sisters' suggestion, I sent Becky a dozen red roses and begged for her forgiveness. She refused to accept my apology. Bipolar disorder had cost me the first of many close friends I would lose throughout my lifetime.

CLINICAL OVERVIEW (CHAPTER ONE)

W*hat are the definition and symptoms of bipolar disorder?*
Bipolar disorder is a mental illness, formerly known as manic depressive disorder, which causes shifts in a person's mood, energy, and ability to function. As the understanding of this disorder has evolved for over a century, the American Psychiatric Association (APA)'s *Diagnostic and Statistical Manual of Mental Disorders: DSM-5* (2013) now dedicates a full chapter to help healthcare professionals diagnose bipolar and related disorders. The chapter was placed after the schizophrenia spectrum and other psychotic disorders, but before depressive   disorder, to designate "a bridge between the two diagnostic classes in terms of symptomology, family history, and genetics"[1].

There are two main types of bipolar disorder: type I and type II, classified according to the severity of mania that an individual experiences. In bipolar I, the individual experiences full-blown mania, "a distinct period of abnormally and persistently elevated, expansive, or irritable mood, and abnormally, and persistently increased goal-directed activity or energy, lasting at least one week and present most of the day, nearly every day"[2]. Those diagnosed with bipolar II experience a milder form of mania, known as hypomania. Individuals with either diagnosis have also experienced at least one major depressive episode before or after the mania or hypomania.

Manic symptoms include a mix of grandiosity, distractibility, extreme participation in pleasure-seeking or risky behavior, decreased need for sleep, excessive talkativeness, racing thoughts, and a rise in goal-directed behavior. The shift in mood is so extreme that it significantly impairs the individual's ability to function occupationally or socially. It often requires hospitalization to prevent harm to self or others. Additionally, losing touch with reality, (also known as psychotic features), can be present. When these symptoms go untreated, they often result in damaged relationships, poor job performance, and even thoughts of suicide or homicide.

Although there is no cure, bipolar disorder can be treated with medication, psychotherapy, and stress reduction. Stress has been known to particularly trigger a bipolar episode in individuals who have a family history of this illness, where the risk of being diagnosed with bipolar syndrome is ten times greater (National Alliance on Mental Illness, 2017).

Each year, 2.9 % or 9.4 million of the U.S. population is diagnosed with bipolar disorder[3]. Many members of society do not understand the symptoms. They can mistake an individual who is experiencing a severe episode as being drunk, drugged, neurotic, crazy, demonized, or even having a brain tumor, as I experienced firsthand.

CHAPTER TWO FIRST EPISODE – PART 2 SUICIDE ATTEMPT

As an amateur songwriter, I composed a song for Becky in an effort to win back her friendship, to no avail. After our incident, she hightailed it out of the building, presumably breaking her lease in the process.

I saw her only once before she left. She was carrying her clothes basket down to the laundry room. I was lugging bags of groceries up the steep stairwell. When she gazed down and saw me approaching, she whirled and raced back upstairs to her apartment. She slammed the door and dead-bolted the lock.

With my best friend now permanently out of my life, I dipped into a deep depression, and began to consider suicide. Being somewhat of a recluse, my few male friends were more or less acquaintances, who were married with children. My own marriage had failed the previous year after seven years of peaks and valleys. Our inability to conceive children was the main culprit in its eventual demise. I felt as though I had no place to turn. My platonic friendship with Becky meant everything to me. My self-destructive thoughts were also clearly being fueled by my bipolar mood swings that had yet to be diagnosed.

The top floor of my building provided immediate access to the roof through an unhinged trapdoor. It was situated in proximity to my third-floor apartment. During the summer months, I would occasionally sunbathe.

I was in the early stages of my first episode and was not fully aware that bipolar disorder's untreated chemical imbalance in my brain was significantly contributing to my clinical depression. Coupled with the loss of Becky, I was contemplating thoughts of returning to my drinking days. An inventory of my liquor cabinet revealed a comprehensive lineup of every alcohol imaginable: rum, bourbon, whiskey, scotch, vodka, gin and tequila.

I strategized my game plan while mixing a lethal concoction of these liquors in an oversized blender. I would climb onto the roof in an inebriated state and gather the courage to hurl myself over the ledge.

Removing the trapdoor, I placed the blender of mixed drinks above me. The commotion must have roused the elderly woman in the apartment adjoining mine. When she stepped out in the hallway and spotted me acting strangely, she tried in vain to discourage me from accessing the roof. I proceeded to elevate myself like a gymnast on a pullup bar onto the flat tar surface. Surveying the surrounding scenery, I saw treetops, telephone wires, and neighboring high-rise apartment buildings.

Grasping the container tightly, I inhaled several gulps of my homemade brew and almost vomited. The potent mixture of alcohol went straight to my head. I swallowed a few more mouthfuls and staggered to the roof's edge and glanced down. After momentarily ignoring my fear of heights, I decided to abandon my attempt. I jerked back and regained my balance. With my equilibrium intact, I returned through the trapdoor to my apartment.

But my suicidal thoughts remained. My plan B was to simply drink myself to death within the comfort of my own home. I would descend into a deep slumber and choke on my own vomit. It would be the most painless and cowardly way to go.

To set the tone, I removed a framed photograph of the Three Stooges from my wall and set it on the kitchen floor. I opened the freezer and pulled out a plastic container of chicken noodle soup that Becky had cooked for me during happier times. It would serve as my last supper and farewell token to her. I warmed it up in the microwave.

I was nude, which seemed to be a recurring theme. Donning my favorite necktie without any reasonable explanation, I rested the pitcher of alcohol on the black and white picture of Curly, Larry, and Moe. After consuming a couple of mighty swigs, I wound up puking all right, except I didn't die as expected. Regrettably, I awoke the following morning with a record-setting hangover.

Later that day, I carried a case filled with my remaining bottles of alcohol and discarded them in the shared basement of our apartment building. I no longer wanted the temptation for new suicidal ideas.

When I returned the following morning to empty my trash, the unopened bottles of liquor had vanished, as I had anticipated if my neighbors discovered them. For many of them, Christmas arrived early that year.

Three Days Later

During my trip to Ireland with a tour group earlier that year while I was still employed by the start-up company, I met Ann Marie, who was spending her summer sightseeing most of Europe. Now in late September, she was planning to cap off her vacation in New England after a brief stopover in New York City. As can be imagined, she had accumulated an incredible amount of souvenirs. Her bag, which had grown to be the size of a small pup tent, was now becoming too cumbersome for any of us who had been on the journey to carry with ease.

That weekend, as decided in advance, I met up with her and a few of our friends from the trip as they were approaching the next-to-last leg of their travels at the World Trade Center. I agreed to babysit the bag for her as they embarked on their final two-week excursion to New England. I would meet them a couple weeks later at the airport before they flew home to England.

I jumped into my car with the oversized fifty-pound duffel bag, and brought it back to my apartment. It wound up being too heavy for me to carry up three flights of stairs. I had a sudden brainstorm.

I drove to my mom's house and lugged the canvas bag to the cellar. As I turned to walk back to my car, I heard my mother and brother scurrying down the stairs to the basement.

"What's this?" asked my mother.

"It's just a harmless bag of souvenirs I agreed to hold for a traveling companion of mine until she returns to New Jersey."

"Oh no, you don't! Get it out of here right now. I don't want it here in my house. It's of the Devil!" She erupted irrationally.

"Where am I going to put it, Mom? There's no place else." My frustration was evident.

"Well then, throw it out. That's what I would do if I were you!"

"I can't just throw it out . . . it doesn't belong to me." I argued, sensing defeat.

Meanwhile, my brother had unzipped the bag and was snooping around. "There's a miniature New York Yankees baseball helmet inside." He remarked suspiciously.

"It's demonic," my mother said.

"Mom, it's a souvenir. She must have picked it up when she was in New York this week for crying out loud!"

"I don't care," my mother said. "I want the bag out of here or I'll throw it out myself."

I was losing ground, but my friend had trusted me with the bag. I had to think quickly. After some deliberation, I managed to drag it into my trunk with my brother's assistance.

Later That Night

I needed a place to store the bag for the next two weeks. I decided to head to my sister Katy's seasonal house in the Poconos.

My father occupied the house year-round as a houseguest. It was a miracle I was able to remember how to get there as I had only driven there a few times, and never late at night like this.

On the way, I stopped by my apartment to get some other belongings I decided to discard. I guess I was beginning to heed my mother and brother's warnings about certain possessions being demonic. I pulled up to a nearby dumpster, and tossed my treasured painting of *The Devil's Coven*, one of only four works I had ever created. For some reason, I also ridded myself of a softball bat. There was no apparent explanation for this, other than it happened to be in my trunk at the time.

Somewhere along the journey, I also dispensed with another of my most valuable possessions: a pair of solid gold cufflinks that I had purchased in Egypt at the Pyramids. They were unique, with my first name encrypted on them in Egyptian letters. However, one of the symbols was a snake, which my brother had convinced me was demonic.

When I arrived at my sister's house at about one a.m., I saw my father through the window in silhouette, sitting in the living room with the lights on. As silently as possible, I dragged the heavy, bulky bag under the wooden porch and brushed some leaves and twigs around it so it wouldn't be noticeable from the street. I knocked on the door. His expression changed to one of horror when he peered through the curtained window and recognized me.

Considering I was his son, it was a bit peculiar that he didn't immediately extend an offer to enter when he cracked the door open. In fairness to him, it must have appeared weird when I flopped down on the couch and blankly stared at him from across the room. I picked up the television remote control and began to fidget with it, acting as if nothing were out of the ordinary. Eventually, his voice broke the silence.

"What are you doing here?" He sounded confused and frightened.

"Oh, I don't know . . . I just decided to go out for a ride," I replied with a bewildered look. "Why? What's the matter? You seem upset."

"You startled me for one thing at this late hour. And I was afraid at first that you might be someone else."

"Like who?"

"There's a strange guy living next door. He never comes out during the day . . . only at night. He never says hello to me. One of the other neighbors told me that they think he is a member of the Witness Protection Program. The government finds places for people like him to live in secluded areas like the Poconos. I heard him earlier taking out his garbage. When he saw me sitting here by the window, he just glared at me. He scares me half to death."

"Well, since I'm up here, why don't you follow me back home to my place and you can stay with me for the night? I just got here, and your story is already starting to give me the creeps."

He reluctantly agreed in light of my own strange behavior.

In retrospect, God was with me again. My excursion wound up being a blessing in disguise. My dad was so unnerved by my unexpected arrival and his scary neighbor, he developed chest pains, which he had checked out. Years earlier, the doctors had surgically corrected three heart valves that were one hundred percent clogged and the fourth one was seventy-five percent blocked. He would now require immediate surgery to install a defibrillator. The surgery was successful and kept him alive for another seven years. If my nocturnal visit hadn't occurred, who knows what might have happened?

My Hospitalization

My own hospitalization was just around the corner, but I wasn't going to go quietly. Shortly before I was admitted to treat my first bipolar episode, one of my neighbors had called the police to complain. She was the same elderly woman who lived in the apartment next to mine, who had tried unsuccessfully to discourage me from climbing up on the roof during my suicide attempt.

Now, I was continuing to be a nuisance as I banged loudly on pots and pans and sang to deafening music during the middle of the day. When the cops arrived, I initially thwarted them by wedging tables, dressers, and the piano in front of the door, and fire escape to block their entry.

"It's the police. Open the door."

"You'll never take me alive, coppers!" I shouted deliriously when I heard their knock.

"Open the door, now!" They banged louder.

Eventually, they coaxed me into allowing them to gain access. They jotted down my information, but then decided not to charge me with disturbing the peace when I calmed my crazy antics. After helping me to move my furniture back to its proper place, they asked me for the phone number of a relative to notify as to what had just occurred.

Shortly thereafter, my sister, Katy, her husband, and other family members, visited my apartment and convinced me I needed hospitalization. They escorted me peacefully to the emergency room in September 1996. I was formally diagnosed with major depression with psychotic symptoms and suicidal ideations. It would be my first of four episodes and hospitalizations being treated for bipolar disorder.

While an inpatient, my entire family came to visit me every day. These bedside gatherings represented a true bonding experience in my life. Initially, some of them had speculated that I had suffered a nervous breakdown, but that notion was quickly dispelled by my doctors.

My sister, Katy, was assigned the duty of cleaning my apartment. She commented on the chicken noodle soup I had splattered on the photograph of The Three Stooges.

"I had to throw out your Three Stooges picture because it looked like you had thrown up spaghetti all over it. I also found five Bibles in your closet. One of them had a pink cover." She seemed startled.

"Oh yeah," I said. "That one was from Mom."

"Where did you get so many Bibles?" she asked.

"Tim and Linda gave the rest of them to me over the years."

I never discovered what Katy did with my Bibles when she took them from my apartment. I didn't even bother to ask, afraid that she would confirm my suspicion that they had been thrown in the garbage. She felt that I had become too religious of late. This would have motivated her to toss them in the trash.

One Week Later

I was discharged from the hospital after a one-week respite. Prior to my release, I was interviewed by a panel of five college students who quizzed me on my bipolar experience. Although I was amenable to the lengthy discussion, it made me feel a bit like a mentally ill guinea pig.

The saga of my friend's souvenir duffel bag had a happy ending. She and her traveling companions returned to town shortly after I finished my hospital stay. I journeyed up to the Poconos and retrieved her belongings, then escorted everyone to the airport as planned, none the wiser.

CLINICAL OVERVIEW (CHAPTER TWO)

W*hat is suicidal ideation and its effect on bipolar disorder?* Individuals with bipolar disorder have a high risk for suicide, especially those who are not in treatment. According to the *Diagnostic and Statistical Manual of Mental Disorders, DSM-5* (2013), people with bipolar disorder have a lifetime risk of suicide fifteen times greater than the general population. This estimate is staggering. The American Psychiatric Association[4] has even cautioned clinicians that one in four completed suicides are related to bipolar disorder.

The American Foundation for Suicide Prevention[5] has reported over one hundred and twenty-one suicides per day in America. Therefore, bipolar disorder likely accounts for approximately thirty daily suicides. Men are three and a half times more likely than women to die by suicide (American Foundation of Suicide Prevention, 2017), and seventy percent of the suicides in 2016 were white males, most of them middle-aged.

Suicidal attempts by those with bipolar disorder usually happen early in the illness, and are almost always triggered by stark depressive or mixed states[6]. For the general public, one in thirty suicide attempts end in death, while for those with bipolar disorder, one in three suicide attempts end in death. This means suicidal attempts for those with bipolar disorder are highly lethal. Furthermore, researchers reported that over thirty-one percent of individuals with bipolar disorder have attempted suicide at least once[7].

Given the high risk of suicide among those with bipolar disorder, there are common warning signs that their loved ones need to be aware of. According to the American Foundation for Suicide Prevention (2016)[8], a change in behavior or completely new behavior is often a red flag, especially if it is associated with a painful experience or loss. Most individuals who commit suicide display one or more warning signs in their talk, behavior, and/or mood. Their conversations might include ideas about them feeling like they are a burden, having no reason to live, feeling trapped, being in pain, and/or contemplating suicide. Their behavior might include isolation, withdrawal, too much or too little sleep, increasing their use of substances, saying goodbye to people, giving away possessions, and an increase in aggression. Their mood might be depressed, irritable, enraged, or anxious. Friends and family should not take these symptoms or changes lightly.

Concerned family members and friends should intervene and get their loved one quickly to a psychiatrist—a medical doctor who specializes in the diagnosis and treatment of mental disorders. Because an imbalance in brain chemicals (known as neurotransmitters) impairs the judgment of a person with bipolar disorder, successful treatment usually requires medicine. Sometimes individuals shy away from psychiatrists because there is still a stigma regarding mental illness; however, psychiatrists are medical doctors with expertise in psychotropic medicine—drugs designed to affect the mind, emotions, and behavior. Primary care physicians are not experts in this field, and because medicine is such an integral part of treatment for those with bipolar disorder, it is wisest to get your loved one to a psychiatrist, psychiatric nurse practitioner, or neurologist as soon as you can.

If the bipolar individual is already under treatment by a psychiatrist (or comparable medical practitioner), call their doctor immediately when you notice such behavior. If they are not under the care of a psychiatrist, take them to a local emergency room, as most hospitals have psychiatrists or other trained mental health practitioners on call to handle mental health crises. If the loved one refuses to go to the hospital, call a suicide hotline or 9-1-1 for assistance. At the writing of this book, the following services were available:

- National Suicide Prevention Hotline: 1-800-273-8255
- Firefighter Behavioral Health Alliance: 1-847-209-8208
- Fire/EMS Helpline: 1-888-731-FIRE (3473)
- Safe Call Now: 1-206-459-3020
- First Responder Assistance Program: 1-855-207-1747
- SAMHSA: 1-800-662-HELP (4357)
- Volunteer Firefighter Alliance: 1-844-550-HERO (4376)
- Crisis Text Line: Text741741

Do not be surprised when people with bipolar disorder lack good judgment and refuse help from those trying to intervene. Chemical imbalance negatively affects the frontal lobe of the brain. The frontal lobe controls one's moral reasoning and good judgment. It is easy to assume that these individuals are manipulative, however, oftentimes they are not in control of these thoughts and rationalizations. They might need family members and/or friends to literally be their frontal lobe accountability partners when their judgment is impaired. Once these individuals' brain chemicals are restored to normal levels, they will not need such an extreme intervention.

Steve West

GROWING UP
BIPOLAR

CHAPTER THREE MY CHILDHOOD DAYS

I was born the fifth of nine children in May 1957. I never met my oldest brother, Bobby. He died four years before my birth. If he had lived, I would never have been born. My parents, devout Roman Catholics, had planned to stop having children after the first three were conceived: Bobby, Jon, and Jamie.

In those days when one attended Catholic school, a doctor would visit each year to perform physicals on the children. In March of 1953, the doctor noted that Bobby's tonsils were very large. He recommended to my parents that they be removed. Bobby was six years old at the time. Heeding his advice, my parents set the surgery date for Good Friday when the schools would be closed.

The tonsils were to be extracted in the doctor's office. The night before the surgery, Bobby woke my mother and said he couldn't sleep, and that there was an angel in his room, beckoning him. My mother thought nothing of it, assuming he was having a dream.

The following morning, with my father in the waiting room, the doctor prepared Bobby for surgery by administering ether. No anesthesiologist was present. Bobby began turning blue and was having trouble breathing. In a panic, the doctor ran out into the waiting room to advise my father, instead of performing the necessary emergency tracheotomy. My father hurried inside the doctor's office and stood by helplessly as Bobby cried out: "Daddy, I'm scared . . . please hold my hand!" Then he passed away.

My father and mother were never the same after that tragedy. My parents, in a state of depression, decided God had punished them for not wanting more children. As a result, they produced six more offspring in a space of ten years.

***

Whenever I played board games as a child with my older siblings, Jon, Jamie, and Marlene, they would always gang up on me. It didn't matter if we played *Risk* or *Monopoly*. Back then, I was the youngest at seven years old, with a nine-year span between Jon and myself, so they were determined to teach me a lesson I'd never forget. Their constant teasing could be unbearable at times.

Well, what I'll never forget was how I always resorted to fits of anger to thwart their mischievous intentions. For example, just when defeat was imminent, I reached over and wiped out the game board. Their eyes widened in horror when they saw it coming, but were unable to stop me.

"Oh, my God, I can't believe you just did that!" my brother, Jon, exclaimed.

"Then maybe next time you'll stop kibitzing."

Meanwhile, my brother, Jamie, hollered to my mother who was in the kitchen: "Mom, Steve's a big hothead . . . he just knocked over the board again!"

"Well then, don't play with him anymore if you know he's like that."

At which point my sister, Marlene, typically started to cry since she realized *she* would be the youngest one in the group if I didn't play. "But Mom, they're going to start picking on me instead."

"That's it. Put away the games and go to your rooms . . . all of you . . . now!"

My parents could be even bigger hotheads than I sometimes was. At least my mother wasn't physical, which is more than I can say about my father from time to time.

My dad was the only television repairman in our small town. After dinner, he toiled away in his basement workshop. My siblings and I raucously played tag upstairs in the living room. My father heard the ceiling boards creaking, and periodically roared at us through the air vents in his booming voice:

"Stop running around up there if you know what's good for you, or else I'm coming up, and you'll be sorry!"

Typically, we heeded his stern advice but, every now and then, we continued to behave like children.

"That's it! I warned you. Here I come!" he bellowed, as he stomped up the stairs.

"Ahhhh!" we screamed in terror. "Dad's coming! Run and hide!"

We scattered for cover, scared out of our collective wits, and the inevitable happened every time . . . one of us would trip or fall behind the rest of the herd, becoming our father's easy prey. Maybe the best way to describe it was to liken it to a scene on the National Geographic's channel featuring a grownup Cheetah hunting down a baby impala. There was no means of escape for the poor victim . . . most often me.

My father was a big man we respected and feared. We respected his authority and feared the back of his hand.

"This is going to hurt me more than it's going to hurt you," he would lie as he mauled me.

And a few bumps and bruises later, he was heading back to his workshop downstairs in the calm after the storm.

When my siblings heard the room had quieted, they popped their heads up from their various hiding places one by one. This sight was reminiscent to the scene in the *Wizard of OZ* where the Munchkins rise from the bushes to confirm the Wicked Witch was dead. "Is he gone?" They wondered aloud in unison.

Truthfully, the bad times outnumbered the good, although my seven siblings and I had each other to fend for one another. They weren't perfect formative years by any stretch of the imagination, but we survived for the better.

I always sensed my father was intimidated by my mother because of her scholastic background. She was the intellectual one, who spoke five languages and had earned her Master's degree. She was also guilty of rubbing his nose in her achievements on many occasions. This naturally provoked my father into his angry moods in such instances. My dad wasn't necessarily book smart; he was street smart, having grown up in a rough neighborhood in Cleveland, Ohio before relocating to New Jersey.

I hate to paint him in an unfavorable light, especially when he's not here to defend himself. I remain convinced that his ongoing mood swings were the result of latent bipolar tendencies. I speak from experience when I talk about how this mental illness can cause fits of anger if not treated properly with medication. As a result, his sudden outbursts were not his fault to an extent. This condition was not diagnosed back then since so little was known or done about maladies such as manic-depression. Even so, he was no saint by any means when it came to volatile temperament.

On one occasion, my older brother, Jamie was involved in an altercation with my father in the dining room after supper. Words were exchanged, and my dad went airborne across the room to confront Jamie, who was on the other side of our wooden table. My father slammed into it with such force, he split the table in two. My brother left home for good shortly thereafter.

Such Stephen King-ish nightmares still haunt me today . . . like the time my father hurled a five-pound statue at my mother from across the dining room during a flare-up. It missed her head by inches, shattering the glass window behind her into a thousand pieces. Ironically, it was a statue of the Blessed Mother!

Somehow, my father always seemed to be cognizant of the boundaries he couldn't cross if he were to avoid winding up in a permanent prison cell. He possessed one enviable asset in this regard: an excellent throwing arm with incredible accuracy. I attribute this talent to his many years as an exceptional softball player.

He needed it when he flung a glass milk bottle in my mother's direction on yet another unexpected occasion. This time it exploded against the wood-paneled wall in our dining room, barely missing her.

Then there was the time my parents attended a church function on a Saturday night. Apparently, alcohol was consumed. The details remain sketchy; however, at some point during the evening my father became suspicious that my mother was flirting with one of the priests. When they arrived home after the event, my oldest brother, Jon spent the remainder of the night fending off my father from hitting her. Seemingly, there was enough dysfunctional childhood fodder within our ranks to feed an army of psychiatrists in the *Twilight Zone*. Yet, despite all the day-to-day violence, the weekends would invariably wind up the same, with my parents playing a competitive, but friendly game of *Scrabble*. My siblings and I would enjoy this brief hiatus from their endless bickering. Sometimes they would even kiss and make up. And all was well . . . until the next outburst of anger. Then the all-too-apparent frightening mood swings of bipolar disorder would be at it again.

Amusingly, one year our local newspaper wrote a feature article on the West clan designating us as the *Family of the Year*. There was also a photograph of the ten members of our family taken in a group shot. I still keep a framed copy of it on my living room end table reminding me of our crazy childhood, which my parents somehow managed to portray as functional to the outside world.

Given my father's uncontrolled temper, my mother must have had nine lives. She passed away from Alzheimer's disease in 2016 at the advanced age of ninety-one. My father lived to be eighty-three. He died back in 2003 as a result of heart failure.

Here's the surprising, possibly even shocking, aspect given all of the negative accounts I have just shared about my father's mostly miserable adult life:

Based on my interpretation of the King James Bible, my father may be in heaven right now. How can that be? He repented for all of his mean-spirited actions that transpired over the course of his lifetime, and he asked God for forgiveness.

He was baptized into the evangelical faith as a born-again Christian during his last seven years on earth. He changed his ways, mellowed with age and became humble. We grew to become friends, and made peace with each other before he died. Unfortunately, the scars still remain from the formative years of my regrettable childhood, and torment me to this very day.

The message is, if my father can be saved, then so can all of us since we all have sinned and fallen short of perfection.

My Grammar School Days
September 1963 to June 1971

Even in childhood, I often suspected I had some type of mental illness. I was always moody and quick-tempered, causing my siblings to nickname me *short-fuse*. I could throw a tantrum as far as I could throw a baseball back then. My nostrils would flare like a wounded bull at the slightest provocation.

Although my bipolar condition might not have fully manifested until I was approaching forty, there were telltale signs of it as far back as I can remember. I was the skinniest kid in school, weighing about eighty-seven pounds after a hearty breakfast. Despite my frailty, and the fact that I wore glasses, it seemed I was always getting in scuffles with kids much tougher than me. Somehow I often rolled over on top of my opponent, claiming victory . . . and possessed the common sense to scurry for cover when defeat was certain.

An early example of my mood swings was in first grade of my Catholic grammar school. My homeroom nun was Sister Lilian Virginia. There was a coveted prize awarded at the end of each school year for the student who exhibited the most exemplary behavior. As I recall, it was an inexpensive pen and pencil set with symbolic value for the child who served as a positive role model to his peers. Sister Lilian Virginia decided I was worthy of this honor for my hard work, diligence, and even-keeled temperament.

The calendar changed, as did the ups and downs of my seesaw battle with mood swings. It was second grade with my new homeroom nun, Sister Ann Josepha. A pudgy kid named Brian Collins sat next to me and was the class clown.

Brian had a *super eraser*, which was a fad back then. It was an oversized pink eraser approximately six inches long that he would use to perform tricks. Once, situating it halfway on the edge of his desk, he whispered to me, "Hey look, Steve . . . swan dive!"

When smacked, the eraser performed an acrobatic aerial descent gone awry and plummeted to the hardwood floor. Naturally, I erupted with laughter and, yes, this caused me to end up getting reprimanded by our teacher. Another time, Brian was performing his signature swan dive for an audience of one. When he pounded on the desktop edge, the eraser went airborne and landed in a cup of water I had on my desk, splattering it everywhere. I almost wet my pants from laughing.

Unfortunately, Sister Ann Josepha did not share my sense of humor.

"That's it, Master West. You seem to think everything is so funny. You can stay after class today and straighten the desks and clap the erasers."

How fitting, I thought . . . clap the *erasers*. In retrospect, it was outside distractions such as Brian Collins that triggered my mood swings throughout my grammar school years. It was a relentless battle of futility. Brian would induce me into bursting out like a punctured balloon filled with laughing gas. I would be the one getting punished.

Finally, the inevitable occurred. My mother was summoned to school to deal with my behavior. Which was I? A serious student or a frivolous one? I was scolded by the nun and later reprimanded by my mom for being perceived as the latter. Understandably, I didn't win the treasured prize that year.

I had journeyed from first to worst in one short year of grammar school due to my sudden mood shifts. I was already beginning to literally laugh in the face of authority, regardless of consequences. This hardly kept with my strict upbringing where I never dared to question my elders. I attributed my springboard behavior at school to a lack of parental role models as a young child.

In third grade, the good/bad cycle resumed. My homeroom teacher that year wasn't a nun. In fact, she would wind up being the only one who didn't fit that mold in my grammar school days. Her name was Miss D'Antonio. She loved me like an adopted son, and it was a case of mutual affection. She was the proverbial polished apple of my eye.

She witnessed my prim and proper behavior, and my exemplary manners on a daily basis. My grades were stratospheric. There were no class clown distractions. Like a world class sprinter, I maintained the inside track to determine who would win the sought-after prize that year. It came down to me and another brownnoser. As I hoped, I crossed the finish line first.

In fourth grade, I was a cellar dweller once again. Initially, I beamed optimism when I discovered my homeroom teacher was Sister Lilian Virginia again. But, like an Ali/Frazier rematch, I was soon down for the count. On this occasion, it wasn't Brian Collins who delivered the knockout punch. In fact, he was conspicuously absent, probably expelled by then.

This time my next-door-neighbor in class was another rotund, jovial kid named Alan Kroc. The poor guy had warts all over his face. I felt genuine sympathy for him. All the other students mocked him and one time even brought him to tears. But boy, was he funny as hell. He would always bother me for cookies. We often played tag in the schoolyard with a few other classmates. The main objective was to stay away from Kroc, or he'd smother you in a bear hug, and it was all over.

The last I heard of him was years later when he was caught robbing a liquor store with a shotgun. This was one more example of how troubled formative years can come back to haunt you. I didn't receive the coveted prize that year either. Alan Kroc's distractions didn't help the cause. In any event, my good/bad streak was intact.

I was back on track in the fifth grade. My nun was Sister Agnes Patrice. She seemed well into her eighties, practically ready to keel over at any moment. But she saw the good in me, which is all that really mattered. Besides, there were no obstacles in my path, no Brian Collins or Alan Kroc to contend with this time around. And without any distractions, I stayed focused. I didn't have any turbulent mood swings. Naturally, I won the treasured prize for the third time in five years.

In sixth grade, the bottom fell out. Again. Her name was Sister Agnes Margarete. We had an early incident that soured our relationship. It was around the stage of my life that I first noticed tendencies toward anger and aggression. On this particular occasion, our class was playing in the schoolyard during our lunchbreak on a wintry day, and Sister Agnes Margarete was the monitor. My rowdy friends and I were throwing snowballs at each other.

She scolded me as she caught me, snowball in hand. "Master West, put down that snowball . . . now!"

I contemplated my choices. My original intent was to toss it at one of my classmates. But the Devil must have gotten into me. I reeled back and aimed it in her direction. My aim was true. As she turned to avoid contact, it nailed her in the back. As one might expect, the result was not good.

My punishment was severe that day. She sadistically had me remove my gloves and hold a piece of ice in each hand for half an hour. To add to my torment, it was freezing outside. I was afraid I would develop frostbite. Meanwhile, I was in full view of my classmates who had returned to class on the second floor. They opened the windows, some of them mocking me. But to some of them, I became an overnight folklore hero for hitting a nun. No, I didn't win the sought-after prize that year.

The seventh grade is a bit of a blur. Despite my excellent memory, I can only remember the first name of my nun, Sister Marcia. It's also entirely possible she had only a single name, similar to Cher or Madonna. I do recall it being a rebellious year for me. I grew my hair long and wore bell-bottomed jeans and wide pink, orange and yellow ties. I continued to question and challenge authority figures. Sadly, my consecutive on/off streak had been broken. I didn't win the prize.

But eighth grade was my crowning achievement. I hit a nun. Again. But this time it wasn't with a snowball. This time it was with my bare hands. It's a long story, but bear with me. My final year of Catholic grammar school was the last roadblock between me and high school. As mentioned, it had been a roller coaster ride through my first seven years of school. My behavior ranged from one extreme of being perceived as an angel who won the prize, to being awarded the notoriety of class clown with my sarcastic sense of humor. My eighth-grade days fell under the latter category.

My homeroom teacher that year was a nun named Sister Robert Therese, who was well over six-feet tall with a bad complexion. I nicknamed her: Attila, the nun. She conducted herself in a stern ominous manner, which featured manly hands as I would soon discover.

She had given us a homework assignment for our English class and I had forgotten to bring it to school. Instead, I had mistakenly left it on my dining room table. So naturally, when she approached me for my essay, I felt it my duty as class clown to respond sarcastically.

"My dog ate it."

"You little omigon (Nun slang.) Put your hands on your desk!"

Whereupon she proceeded to promptly whack my knuckles with her yardstick. I groaned in agony as she barked at me to go to the front of the room and write my name on the blackboard for detention purposes.

Honestly, I figured she was letting me off easy since the typical punishment in those days was to force you to write one hundred times: "I must not forget my homework." This was usually followed by an order to clap all erasers out on the fire escape, straighten the desks and, of course, empty the waste paper baskets.

My hands were still stinging in pain when I reached the front of the classroom, so I angrily picked up a piece of chalk and scribbled my name on the board. I slammed the chalk down on the ledge as my classmates howled with laughter.

"Why, you little whippersnapper," she cried as she snuck up from behind me.

She yanked my long hair backwards causing me once again to yelp in pain.

"Ow! That really hurt!" I squealed, as I turned to confront her.

But she wasn't finished yet. She slammed the back of my head against the blackboard. In retrospect, it makes me wonder if she also suffered from bipolar disorder.

Feeling understandably shaken, I lunged at her with my face flushed in fury. She extended her arms and came at me to place me into a chokehold. I summoned all my strength and swung mightily with my clenched fist and connected. I gave her a direct shot into her white bib, which disengaged from her black habit and went sailing across the room.

My classmates sat there stunned. It was surreal. Sister Robert Therese set out to retrieve her bib.

Mother Superior was quickly summoned to the scene and the recommended outcome of this ordeal was to have me expelled from school. The Monsignor, who headed the parish and the high school, agreed. It was determined I was not fit to graduate because of this unprecedented encounter with a holy nun.

My mother was instructed to come to school immediately to get me. When she arrived, her Italian blood boiled.

"Is it true you hit a nun, Steve?" She asked, glaring at me.

"Yes! But she hit me first, Mom, so it was self-defense."

At which point, my mother whirled and faced the Monsignor, Sister Robert Therese, Mother Superior, the Vice-Principal, and a swelling crowd that had gathered in the hallway. This included the janitors, and other teachers. She boldly announced, "If anyone, and I do mean anyone, ever hits my son again, I'll come back here and hit them myself!"

Whereupon, everyone stared at the ground sheepishly. Soon the crowd dispersed.

I left early that day and headed home with my mother. I did finish grammar school and continue my high school education in this Catholic Parish. However, eventually when they raised the tuition, I wound up graduating from the local public high school instead.

CLINICAL OVERVIEW (CHAPTER THREE)

*I*s there a link between early childhood trauma and bipolar disorder?

According to the American Psychiatric Association's (APA's) *Diagnostic and Statistical Manual of Mental Disorders: DSM-5* (2013)[9], Bipolar I occurs throughout the lifecycle, even as late as seventy years old. However, eighteen is the mean age when mania, hypomania, or major depression is first experienced. Because the average age is so young, bipolar I symptoms initially surface in many individuals when they are children. Mental health professionals cannot precisely define what is "normal" for each child. Consequently, diagnosing bipolar in children is more complex, and it requires doctors to rely on the youth's unique baseline to properly assess for pediatric bipolar.

The American Academy of Child and Adolescent Psychiatry (AACAP, 2015)[10] reports that bipolar is the outcome of diverse reasons. However, APA (2013) emphasizes that the most compelling and reliable predictor for bipolar is genetics. Adults with a family history of bipolar I or II are ten times more vulnerable for this illness than those without a biological connection. Additionally, research and clinical experience confirms that bipolar disorder can be triggered by trauma or stress in individuals with a genetic predisposition.

Relevant studies indicate that individuals who experience early traumatic life events are at risk of developing bipolar disorders and of having stark clinical presentations of this illness over time[11]. Childhood distress harmfully affects physiology, which in turn negatively alters the ability to regulate affect, control impulses, and function cognitively. Furthermore, the child's ability to later manage adult life stressors is compromised. This suggests that mental health professionals should systematically evaluate the early life trauma of patients with bipolar disorders, especially those with a severe clinical presentation of the diagnosis.

Although there is currently no cure for bipolar disorder, the National Institute of Mental Health (2015)[12] explained that doctors often address pediatric bipolar in the same way they treat adults with this diagnosis. The usual treatment protocol includes a combination of medication and talk therapy. For pediatric bipolar, it is especially helpful when the parents and other family members are educated about the illness and collaborate with the treatment process.

*I*s the diagnosis of bipolar disorder different in children and adults?

As mentioned, The American Psychiatric Association's (APA's) *Diagnostic and Statistical Manual of Mental Disorders: DSM-5* (2013) has explained that the average age of the first manic or major depressive episode is approximately eighteen years old. However, when diagnosing bipolar disorder in children, the APA (2013) has cautioned professionals that special considerations are needed, because it is common for children of the same chronological age to be at different developmental stages. As a result, it is not easy at any point in a child's life for a professional to define what is "normal" or "expected." The APA (2013) has therefore suggested that each child should be judged according to his or her own baseline that is supported by people who know the youth best.

Although the primary feature of a manic episode is a distinct period of abnormally elevated mood, the symptoms may be different in children. For example, the APA (2013) has clarified that goofiness or silliness in children is normal when in the context of a special occasion. However, when these symptoms are inappropriate to context (e.g. such as at school during teaching time), these symptoms may meet the manic criteria. If the silliness is not usual for the child's baseline, and this mood change occurs when there are other symptoms (such as inflated self-esteem, racing thoughts, more talkativeness, distractibility, involvement in activities with probable painful consequences), then this combination may meet the criteria for mania.

When diagnosing a major depressive episode in youth, the APA (2013) has warned clinicians that children might exhibit irritability instead of depression. They also have cautioned mental health professionals that instead of weight loss or gain that is often exhibited in adult depression, with children it might be their failure to meet expected weight gains.

Prior to 2013, when APA published its 5th edition of their *Diagnostic and Statistical Manual of Mental Disorders: (DSM-5)*, mental health practitioners were concerned about an over diagnosis of and treatment for bipolar disorder in children. Therefore, in their 5th edition, the APA identified a new diagnosis to address the presentation of recurring irritability and many behavioral dyscontrol episodes. This diagnosis is known as disruptive mood dysregulation disorder, and it has been added to the depressive disorders for children up to twelve years old. The APA (2013) has asserted that youth who exhibit such a symptom pattern usually develop unipolar depression or anxiety disorders rather than bipolar disorder.

CHAPTER FOUR YOUNG ADULTHOOD

When I switched to the local public high school, I experienced the shock of my life. I had transferred from the strict ways of domineering nuns equipped with yardstick weaponry, to a mindset where anything goes. For an inhibited kid like me, who had been reared by disciplinarian parents and then passed along to overbearing authority figures at school, this was paradise. Temptation was everywhere. Not all of it was healthy.

In 1974, early in my junior year at North Arlington High School, I tried desperately to fit in with my new classmates, but I was painfully shy. One of my sisters, Katy, who had made the same transition the previous year, was doing her best to help me.

I wore my hair down to my shoulders and dressed in the same jeans every day. I was welcome in the hippie crowd who invited me into their fold. I was also a good softball player, which drew some interest from the jocks, who needed a right-fielder. As for me, I wanted to please everyone.

Mario, a fellow sophomore of Katy's was hosting a huge party one weekend at his parents' house while they were out of town. Katy got me an invitation in an effort to make new friends, both in her grade and mine. Katy was very popular in school and much more outgoing than I was.

Saturday night arrived, and I hooked up with my very first drinking buddy at that party. His name was Blackberry Brandy. The two of us had never met before, but we had an instant connection. Aside from a few bottles of beer that my older sister Marlene had bought for me, I had never had more than a sip of alcohol in my life. Nevertheless, I decided to go big that night, and foolishly consumed the whole bottle within a few hours.

I had eaten a hearty dinner before the party, including spinach and beets. About three hours into the wild bash, these vegetables made a second appearance—flying through the living room. The bulk of it landed between the cushions of Mario's parents' expensive couch, sending partygoers scattering for cover.

In retrospect, the others might have also been afraid of Mario's renowned temper, and worried I would become the target of his anger. He played on the high school varsity football team and was a known aggressive player. I weighed about one hundred and seventeen pounds back then, and that's with a bottle of beer in each pocket.

Thankfully, my sister Katy intervened. Ben, another friend of hers, escorted me outside for fresh air until I was finally finished vomiting. He told me to wait on the front porch for him while he said his goodbyes. The game plan was for him to take me home per my sister's instructions to ensure I arrived safely.

I grew impatient and started stumbling around, looking for a place to relieve my bladder in some nearby hedges. As I was unzipping, I tripped and fell into the bushes. After what seemed like an eternity, I was able to right myself. In my inebriated state, I headed back to Mario's house in the wrong direction. Soon I was totally lost and there was no sign of Ben.

Oblivious, I staggered up to Mario's neighbors' front porch steps, ringing their doorbells and asking them if they knew where 'Mario' lived. I received mixed reactions of anger, fright, and shock. One of the neighbors must have called the police, as only moments later, cops arrived on the scene with their red and blue lights flashing.

They asked me my name and where I resided. (I lived on Canterbury Avenue at the time.) So, I responded, "I'm Deve Swest and I live on Blackberry Avenue." I struggled to maintain my balance.

"All right, let's take him home," one of the officers said once they had managed to somehow confirm my real street address.

"You're not going to get sick again are you?" They inquired as they loaded me into the back seat. There were telltale signs of vomit on my clothes and on my breath.

"No, I'm fine, Obcifer." I hiccupped as I slumped down. I only lived on the other side of the small town, which was maybe a mile away. It may have been a sudden bump in the road that jarred it loose, but suddenly, and without warning, I had this unstoppable urge to hurl. Once again, my spinach and beets went soaring, this time directly on the seat next to me, right into the officers' hats.

"Ahh, don't tell me you just did what I think you did?" groaned one of the cops.

I nodded as I wiped my lips with my shirt sleeve.

"You little son of a bitch!" he bellowed.

We soon arrived at my house, and they carried me to the side door foyer and rang the bell. When my mother swung the door open, I fell forward and landed facedown with a thud on the kitchen floor.

"Who did this to you?" she demanded of me in her naiveté.

Even in my inebriated stupor, I retained enough common sense to blame it on my sister's friend, Ben. My mother never entirely forgave him for that episode. Along with one of my younger sisters, Vicki, my mother stayed up with me all night, worried I would puke in my sleep and choke on my own vomit.

We experienced a small kitchen fire the very next night. Flames from one of the stove burners caught the nearby blinds on fire. We were able to douse the minor blaze quickly, but we called the cops as a precaution.

Who arrived at our kitchen doorstep, but the very same two policemen from the night before. When our eyes met, they growled at me in unison. I returned the scowl, not even trying to conceal my disdain for authority figures. They were both wearing their hats, and I chuckled at the thought of them washing them out because of me.

Summer 1975

The next step in my escape from reality was to graduate from alcohol to marijuana. The first time I smoked pot, I was driving down the Jersey shore with Tina, one of the most popular girls in our small hometown. We were traveling south on the Garden State Parkway in my recently purchased, used 1971 Chevy Nova. I was on top of the world.

To what did I owe my good fortune? My sudden allure was due to me being one of the only guys in town with a car. Besides, Tina and I were just friends, and I was chauffeuring her for a weekend visit with her steady boyfriend.

In return for my personal limo service and good company, she provided the weed. We smoked two joints. One was already overkill since I had built up zero immunity to inhaling this foreign substance. Tina and I began chuckling for no apparent reason. Any words uttered by either one of us resulted in heightened hysteria. Suddenly we were both hungry and needed something to snack on.

I noticed that we also needed gas, so I pulled into a station in a rest area. There were dozens of dead mosquitoes on my windshield, and I was out of wiper fluid. The musclebound attendant was in his early twenties, and he approached my driver's side and inquired the expected, "What can I getcha?"

Tina began giggling increasingly louder.

"Fill it up, regular," I replied, biting my lip to control my unwarranted laughter. "Oh, and can you clean my windshield, please?" I gestured at the flattened mosquitoes. "It's all mushy."

Tina roared liked a lion with delight at this silly remark and I, uncontrollably, followed suit. The bulky attendant thought we were making fun of him. "What are you— a fucking asshole, pal?" he snarled.

Fearing for our lives, I bolted without purchasing any gas at that stop. The dead mosquitoes remained with us as well. Fortunately, by the time we reached the next rest area, Tina and I had both descended from our high. I filled the tank, and the attendant squeegeed my windshield, removing the deceased insects. We lived to see another day.

Autumn 1975

Unfortunately, my experiences involving alcohol and drugs at school did not all end favorably. Arguably, one of the biggest mistakes and poorest decisions I have ever made in my life, was when I was eighteen years old and a senior in high school. That was the night I allowed two of my so-called friends, Andy and Josh, to persuade me into dropping a hit of LSD in the form of blotter acid. It was such a tiny strip of substance that it appeared harmless when it dissolved on my tongue in a matter of seconds.

Except a short while later, I embarked on a terrifying trip. In retrospect, it reminds me of a bipolar episode, only without the mania part. I sometimes wonder with regret if destroying my brain cells with this trip played a role in causing the chemical imbalance that contributed to my future bouts of bipolar. The sensation was a hallucinatory fireball that left my brain totally fried. I was never so paranoid in my life, convinced that everyone was out to get me. In a sense, it wasn't far from the truth.

We started with a drive to the county park where we consumed some Miller beers and met up with a few other buddies who were also tripping. The group of us smoked a joint or two for good measure. I was seeing *trails* at the time, and it appeared as if everyone was moving in slow motion.

Andy and Josh drove me to the house of one of our fellow classmates, Dick, who apparently had a sadistic sense of humor. I sat down on the couch in the corner of the living room. This guy had a nasty German shepherd barking up a storm in his bedroom. When Dick opened the door, the dog sprang forward in my direction. Dick pointed at me with a horrific smile and said, "Sic him, boy!"

I saw trails of a dozen German shepherds launching toward me. I cowered into a protective fetal position and pleaded for mercy. Dick, enjoying my torment, instructed his dog to retreat. But the worst was yet to come, and my friends looked on and said nothing.

Dick removed a shotgun from the shelf above his head and placed it in his lap. He pretended to load shells into it as I would later discover laughing the entire time. Then he arose and sat down alongside me on the couch. He slowly placed the shotgun against the side of my head. I thought for sure I would die. Then I heard the click as he pulled the trigger once and hollered.

"Bang!"

I freaked out as I realized he hadn't loaded the gun. I prayed to God that my trip to hell would end soon. I finally did survive the journey, but I left three lost souls behind in the flames. The next morning I lay curled in a ball in the corner of my bedroom, crying like a baby.

Never again. Period.

My Brother's Death

In January 1983, I was twenty-five years old when tragedy struck the West household. Our second oldest brother, Jon, who had hypertension since childhood, was driving home from his job at IBM. He was thirty-four years old. He had recently been promoted to director and, as we learned later, his prescribed meds were making him sluggish, so he occasionally stopped taking them.

Several eyewitness accounts reported he had just driven through the toll booth in Cornwall, New York, when his car veered off into the median and subsequently a drainage ditch. Fellow motorists tried to revive him but he was already dead from an apparent heart attack.

I got the call from my youngest sister, Linda at one o'clock in the morning. When the phone rings at that hour, it is never good news. This was no exception.

In an unusually calm voice, she said, "Steve, Jon's dead. They think he was killed in a car accident."

"Jon who? Jon who?" I was in a state of shock.

"Jon, our brother."

"Are they sure?"

"Yes, Steve. Jon is dead." She sounded agitated with me.

I put on two winter coats that January night as I began to shiver uncontrollably after the call.

We agreed that all the siblings would meet at our mother's house to tell her the terrible news. When we arrived, my oldest sister Marlene awakened her from a deep sleep and told her as gently as possible. We all took turns consoling her throughout the night. For days upon weeks without end, my mother just sat in her rocking chair staring out the window in stunned disbelief, saying nothing.

For my siblings and me, the death of our oldest brother and leader marked the end of childhood innocence.

My Marriage September 1987 – March 1995

I met my wife Diane in 1986 through a singles classified ad I placed in a New Jersey monthly magazine. My blind dates had been one disaster after another so I figured I would try a new approach to meeting someone. My friends were all getting married and suddenly I was in a rush to tie the knot. I can't recall my exact words in the ad, but I do remember the corny ending was something to the effect of ". . . seeking a love story that ends with happily ever after." I must have received fifty responses. Most of them included photographs with their letters. I chose Diane because I found her to be physically attractive. She was tall and thin with short brown hair and blue eyes. She also appeared to have a wacky sense of humor; she asked me in her letter if I was an axe murderer. I was thirty when we married a year later, Diane a year younger. Right away, there were indications that things were not as they appeared to be, but I chose to ignore them. For example, why was such a beautiful woman still on the market at her age?

In any event, 1986 was the year the Mets won the World Series. We would sit on the couch each night devouring popcorn and washing it down with a pitcher of Sangria that had become my specialty.

She knew all the players' names: Dwight Gooden, Gary Carter, Keith Hernandez, Mookie Wilson, Lenny Dykstra and, of course, Daryl Strawberry. She had me convinced she was the world's biggest baseball fan. Wow, I thought, a woman who loves sports, what a dream come true.

The season passed and we were married the following year. One night I asked her to turn on the television because the Mets game was about to begin. "Put a bag of popcorn in the microwave," I said, "and I'll make a pitcher of Sangria."

She stared at me with a blank expression and said. "Steve, I hate baseball." Then she turned and went into the bedroom, shutting the door behind her.

My jaw dropped like a misplayed fly ball as it dawned on me. She had waited to get the ring on her finger before showing her true feelings.

There were other indicators as well. For instance, just prior to our wedding, I wrote two love songs for her. One of them was a ballad which I had hoped we could choose as our wedding song. It was called "Song for Diane."

I took her to the recording studio one night to hear the songs, and afterwards asked her, "Well, what do you think? Do you like them?"

She gave no response. My heart was broken. We wound up dancing to a lame pop song at our wedding called "Always," instead of the personal song I had recorded. Why hadn't I noticed these obvious signs? Was I that desperate to get married?

As we began to feel more comfortable with each other, the fighting started. Our anger continued to escalate. One morning, after a heated exchange, she stormed out of the house on her way to work. She slammed the front door behind her with such force that our wedding picture came crashing off the wall. How fitting, I thought.

A big part of her frustration came from our repeated attempts to conceive a baby. We tried everything, from artificial insemination to in vitro fertilization, without success. She had two operations to have her fallopian tubes scraped. I learned new words like endometriosis. She blamed me for having a low sperm count, and even accused me of not wanting to have a baby.

To make the most of an unpleasant situation, I tried to get her to travel the world with me. We journeyed to every country in Western Europe. We visited Rio de Janeiro for Carnival, the Orient, and Hawaii as part of our honeymoon. At times, she appeared to be happy. Other times, she was reluctant to join me.

We experienced a glimmer of hope one month when her period was late. She was ecstatic that she might be pregnant and even shared the potential good news with her sister. I tended to be cautiously optimistic before becoming too excited. It wasn't long after that I came home one night and found her lying face down in bed crying into her pillow. After that incident, our marriage continued on a rapid descent.

She stayed late at her job several times a week, burying herself in her work. I played in tennis and softball leagues, two or three times a week as well. When I returned home after joining my friends for beers and showered, it was around ten o'clock. Most of the time she still wasn't home. At first, I just assumed she was having an affair, and maybe she was, who knows? The crazy part was when I would call her at work at that incredibly late hour, guess what? She would answer her phone on the first ring! "Hello, Pricing," which was the name of her department.

My anger was beginning to escalate to a level that I would later recognize as latent bipolar disorder. For instance, one Sunday afternoon I decided to chop down a twenty-five foot maple tree in our backyard whose roots were interfering with our aboveground pool. The fact that I chose to perform this task on a whim most likely suggested a bit of mania was developing. I am typically not known for my handyman prowess and had never attempted such a feat before. I climbed a ladder and was able to remove many of the uppermost branches with a trimmer. When it was time to bring the tree down, I alternated between a chainsaw and a good old-fashioned axe.

I had secured a rope in strategic places since there was a very small margin for error to prevent it from landing in our pool. The alternative outcome would have been far worse. It could have crashed through the roof of our house. The third and obvious most tragic occurrence would have been to have it land on my wife or myself, in which case I wouldn't be writing this story. But, there was no turning back.

Why hadn't I hired a professional? I also later found out I should have had a town permit to remove the tree. I hacked at the remaining stump while my wife tugged on the rope to guide it toward a safe landing spot. Blisters blossomed on my hands as I gripped the axe. At one point, my wife chided me into hurrying since she was growing weary of pulling on the rope.

I growled at her. "Shut up or I'll chop you down!"

I began to shudder. What had become of me? Had those words really come from my mouth? I later apologized, but the emotional damage was done. She said nothing in return.

Through our joint efforts, we successfully removed the tree. Unfortunately, it would be one of our last acts together. Shortly thereafter, I asked her for a divorce. Although I had never cheated on my wife, I was facing temptation, so I knew it was time to quit.

She suggested we see a marriage counselor to mend our relationship. I was hesitant, but I eventually agreed to attend one session. The counselor was a middle-aged woman sporting a red fashion scarf.

"You can go first," I said to Diane.

She came out swinging and startled me. "I would have given my left arm to have a baby, but Steve never wanted to have one! And when we went on vacation, we always went where he wanted to go. He never cared about me!" She went on and on, voice cracking.

I was genuinely shaken up and hurt to hear these harsh and untrue words come from the woman I once thought I loved. All our magnificent vacations . . . we had just returned from Scandinavia. We had accumulated a lifetime of memories in seven short years. Suddenly I felt so empty inside.

As far as the baby was concerned, I thought of all the trials we had endured. She was accusing me of not showing any care or emotion. Even the counselor was surprised at Diane's eruption and cautioned her.

"Diane, in my profession, it's my responsibility to be objective. However, I think your husband is right. There is another side to the story that you need to consider if you hope to make a relationship successful."

But, I already knew it was too late to turn back. She had been deceiving me from the onset. Our marriage was over. In the car on the way home, Diane was still livid.

"I just wanted to take that woman's red scarf and strangle her with it!"

In retrospect, there may have been a bit of bipolar disorder in both of us. Mine finally surfaced a short while after our divorce. I reached out to her only once more a few years later unsuccessfully. I had found hundreds of photographs of her family in some old albums that I thought she would cherish. However, I was able to touch base with her older brother. He shared tragic news with me about their family. Diane's sister Joyce had recently died of breast cancer, and her seventeen-year-old nephew, Eric had been killed in a car accident. I felt genuinely upset since I had gotten to know Joyce and Eric quite well during our seven years together.

From time to time, I still think about our failed marriage. I sincerely wish Diane well, and hope she found true happiness.

My Severe Mood Swings (Workplace – 1993)

A few years before losing my job and having my first manifestation of bipolar disorder, I started experiencing mood swings at work. I was the account manager none of the support staff wanted to work with. Every year, the company switched my sales team to try to improve this uncomfortable situation. I was nice to my coworkers as a member of the company's softball team, and we often enjoyed a postgame bar visit to shoot pool and throw darts. But I was painfully difficult to be around during the workday.

On one occasion, during an argument with one of my colleagues, he cruelly blurted out, "Nobody likes you!"

This statement seemed to echo the sentiments of the rest of my fellow workers, but not our customers or vendors, who always seemed to like me. I was somehow able to control my mood swings when the setting called for it.

My biggest problem was undoubtedly handling stress. I would later realize this was often a trigger for my bipolar episodes. Perhaps the worst possible occupation for pressure-filled situations is sales, the occupation I had inexplicably chosen.

The following example illustrates my inability to operate effectively under duress. Larry was my administrative assistant, and Norman served as my technical backup. We had a proposal deadline, and Larry was late in relaying the pricing information. I was sitting in my cubicle discussing the situation with Norman and becoming increasingly irate with Larry's tardiness.

I dialed Larry's extension and ordered him to join us immediately. He arrived moments later holding paperwork, which I assumed was the needed documentation.

"Give me that!" I leapt from my chair and snatched the papers from him. "What took you so long?" My nostrils flared.

Norman tried to intervene, but it was too late. Larry lurched forward and pointed his finger against my nose. "Don't you ever do that again or I'll kill you, West!" Then he stormed back to his desk.

Steve West

Pretty strong talk for someone who professes to be a born-again Christian, I thought. But, then again, I wasn't exactly creating an exemplary perception myself. I called Larry later to apologize, but he let the call go to voice mail. His greeting ended with the somewhat predictable, "Have a *blessed* day." Hypocrite.

On the Dating Scene Singles Cruise – 1993

My moodiness spilled over into the dating scene, both with women I worked with at the office and those I met after hours. It seemed as if the pattern was always the same. At first, they found me physically attractive, and complimented me on being a nice guy. But they would inevitably lose interest because I was too moody, especially when I drank.

The truth is, I've always been somewhat shy around women, so I invariably found myself turning to the great equalizer: alcohol.

At one particular juncture, albeit a short one, I considered myself to be "a problem drinker." I joined my friends after hours at the bar dozens of times. If I were late for the gathering, I would simply double up on my drinks to catch up with my buddies. Eventually, this caught up with me in the form of my unfortunate DWI incident later in 1993.

I especially abused alcohol when away on vacation, such as the six or seven singles cruises I embarked on over the years. One trip that stands out is a voyage to the Grand Cayman Islands and Ocho Rios, Jamaica. There were about twenty-five of us on the excursion, mostly women, so it seemed I had my choice. There was one I was mildly interested in (I tended to be picky). Her name was Karen. As the night progressed, she appeared to have her eyes on me as well.

I consumed a half dozen rum and cokes just to ask her to dance and another six to gather the courage to invite her up to my cabin. She said

66

yes. It was only then I remembered I had a roommate, and it was past two o'clock in the morning. When I selfishly rustled him out of bed at that ungodly hour, he surprisingly complied and granted us a half hour as he stood in the hall outside of our cabin in his pajamas.

It turned out it wasn't necessary. I passed out on the bed only moments after entering the room. Karen took my inebriated inactions as a sign of disinterest, and was livid. She avoided me for the remainder of the cruise.

My DWI Car Accident

I had a few drinks . . . then had a few more. I grabbed my car keys and headed out the door that ill-fated night of November 19, 1993. I had been celebrating the promotion of one of my colleagues at a hotel bar and drinking on an empty stomach. My house was southeast of the hotel. In my inebriated state, I headed home in a northwest direction onto Route 80 west.

Driving aimlessly, I got off at an exit approximately twenty miles away. Soon I was on a winding, single lane road heading to the middle of nowhere. As the hour approached midnight, it began to rain. Hypnotized by my windshield wipers swaying back and forth, I felt myself starting to nod. I turned up the volume on my *Graceland* CD, Paul Simon's recent number one hit. I rolled down the window to let in the cold air in a desperate attempt to fight off my increasing weariness.

The last thing I remembered in my semi-subconscious state was the solitary sound of BOOM! I thought I woke up dead. Instead, there were paramedics trying to rip open my driver's side door with the Jaws of Life. The airbag in my new car had apparently saved my life. A young woman and a girl sat huddled under a blanket in the rain on the side of the road as the paramedics prepared to load me into the ambulance. My glasses lay shattered at my feet on the floor of my demolished car.

Through several eyewitness accounts and the police report, I learned later what had happened. Traveling at forty miles an hour, I had drifted into the lane of oncoming traffic and caused a head-on collision with a small pickup truck. There was a young man driving the vehicle, along with his wife, who was five months pregnant, and their nine-year-old niece. They had no time to swerve.

The force of the impact was staggering since I wasn't braking. I sent their truck soaring approximately thirty feet backwards. It landed with its back tires spinning over the side of the guardrail overlooking a rocky ravine. The police report estimated that had I knocked them back any further, their truck would have toppled over the bridge, killing them all.

The officer at the hospital explained that had that happened I would have been arrested on multiple charges of vehicular manslaughter while intoxicated. This was a charge carrying a potential sentence of fifteen years . . . fifteen years along with the horrifying knowledge I had taken four innocent lives. I would essentially lose mine as well if I wound up spending the prime of my life behind bars.

There's no doubt in my mind I should have died that night. I genuinely believe a guardian angel was watching over me and giving me a second chance to avoid spending eternity in hell. I learned my lesson loud and clear. To this day, twenty-five years later, I haven't taken even a sip of alcohol then gotten behind the wheel.

I did tear the PCL ligament in my left knee when it slammed against the dashboard, but, amazingly suffered no broken bones. Even more astonishing was the fact the other driver sustained only a broken ankle. There were no other injuries including to the unborn fetus. Of course, there was the terrible emotional anguish I had put them through. The accident occurred in the town of Hope, a place I had never been before.

I lost my license for seven months, which was a small price to pay considering the circumstances. My employer told me they would not fire me, but it was understandably my responsibility to make it into work each day. Since I lived twenty-five miles from the office, this posed a major problem. I frantically searched the classifieds for lodging and found the only place within walking distance of my office was a rundown boarding house.

Humbling myself, I spent the next seven months living with ten derelicts on welfare. This was during one of New Jersey's snowiest winters on record. The snow was so deep on the sidewalks I had to trudge to work in the middle of the street, dodging traffic each day.

I was in the middle of my divorce, which was one of the reasons I had developed a drinking problem. As part of the settlement, I was trying to sell our house which I finally did, commuting back and forth by taxi from the boarding house on weekends to our home to meet with prospective buyers and the realtor. In my desperation, I accepted an offer twenty thousand dollars below market value.

I struggled through the seven months until my license was reinstated. But even with my newfound joy, I couldn't forget that rainy night in the town of Hope. The fate of four innocent strangers and mine were left hanging in the balance—between life and death, freedom and prison, heaven and hell, for eternity. Eternity. I couldn't believe how close tragedy had been.

Australia – 1995 and 1997

I have been fortunate to visit Australia on three occasions. The first time was in 1983 when I was recovering from my brother's death. That was long before my bipolar disorder fully manifested in 1996.

My second excursion down under occurred in early 1995 as my mood swings were worsening, predictably in the presence of alcohol.

I was in a dive bar in the middle of The Outback, feeling no pain as I danced on top of a pool table holding a bottle of Triple XXX beer. My other fist was pumping wildly into the air. I was belting out a tune from the local band "Men at Work." Accompanying me were two attractive Sheilas on either side: Joanne to the left and Sharon to the right. And, in case that isn't enough of a visual, I was dressed in drag. Yes, just slightly out of character for me.

Liquored up, I was the life of the party, but in the morning, I sulked at the tiniest provocation, sensing something was wrong. But I equated it simply to being hungover from the night before.

My recurring mood swings dampened the atmosphere on our bus tour on a daily basis particularly since I was the senior member of a group comprised of teenagers and young adults. They looked up to me as somewhat of a fatherly figure. Fortunately, I would "snap out of my funk" as the new day progressed. I would apologize and return to my jovial self and things would revert to normal until the next time.

In 1996, when I entered the dark, tangled labyrinth of bipolar disorder, my life would never be the same. My first of four episodes was the catalyst to partially impact the next fifteen years of my life. In retrospect, the decades of my forties and early fifties amounted to one colossal blurred memory. Thirty-five photo albums, containing more than eleven thousand snapshots taken over these years, serve as some of my only reminders of those stolen days.

In 1997 I returned a final time to Australia to renew some old acquaintances, and explore faraway places such as Sydney, Melbourne, Perth, and Tasmania. Later, I recorded four songs at the studio in a tribute to my favorite continent. This trip was my fondest of my three Australian excursions. I had eliminated alcohol from my repertoire and was enjoying life sober, with the exception of a wine tasting in Adelaide, South Australia.

On the Sports Front

I had always been a huge sports fanatic, who played in softball and tennis leagues for the better part of twenty years. Typically the leadoff batter on my softball team, I was an excellent singles and doubles hitter, who had a propensity to get on base. However, in the aftermath of my first bipolar episode, I often stood like a statue at the plate unable to get the bat off my shoulder. The best I could manage were line drives back to the pitcher, and I even struck out once or twice, which is a difficult feat in slow-pitch. My hand-to-eye coordination was shot. In retrospect, this was most likely a result of being overly-medicated during my initial episode. Eventually, I was moved from the leadoff position down to the final slot in the batting order. I quit the team at the end of the season and gave up the sport for good.

I had also been wearing a sports brace to compensate for the PCL ligament torn in my left knee during the car accident several years earlier. The cumbersome contraption often slid down my leg and had to be constantly adjusted.

Concerning tennis, I had won the first place trophy on multiple occasions against suitable competition at my level. After my initial bipolar episode my game diminished so poorly that I had difficulty finding a beatable opponent. One night, I played the lowest-ranked member in our league. During our one-hour session, he destroyed me—shutting me out completely. I barely returned any of his lob shots and was hardly able to make contact with the ball. I was moving in slow motion. He beat me in straight sets; I didn't score a point. After that embarrassing debacle, I discarded my tennis racket as well. My sports career was officially over.

Steve West

CLINICAL OVERVIEW (CHAPTER FOUR)

*I*s *there a link between alcohol/drug abuse and the treatment of bipolar disorder?*
   Bipolar disorder (BD) and alcoholism commonly coincide. The nature of the relationship between these two maladies is complex and not well understood. It appears alcohol use may worsen the clinical course of BD, making it harder to treat. There is also evidence to support a genetic link between the two conditions. BD, complicated by alcoholism, is associated with an increased number of hospitalizations, additional mixed episodes, an earlier age of onset of BD, and more suicidal ideation. Given the prevalence and morbidity of these two disorders, it is important to screen for substance abuse in all bipolar patients and to address it aggressively. Some studies have suggested mood stabilizers may be helpful in treating alcoholic BD patients. However, other studies are needed to address the interactions between these two illnesses which, if not treated, can worsen the course of both conditions[13].

A 2006 *Journal of Substance Abuse Treatment* [14] article found that mood disorders are present in forty to forty-two percent of co-occurring mental health and substance use disorders. While many people abuse drugs to suppress symptoms of BD, the *Diagnostic and*

Statistical Manual of Mental Disorders: DSM-5 (2013)[15] notes that drug use can also induce bipolar symptoms.

Newer research suggests that substance-induced psychosis, especially from marijuana, is significantly linked with later development of both BD and schizophrenia. In a study of almost six thousand and eight hundred patients in Denmark[16] who experienced psychosis induced by any type of substance, about one third developed either schizophrenia or BD within twenty years of follow-up.

According to statistics presented by the American Journal of Managed Care[17],

- About fifty-six percent of individuals with BD who participated in a national study had experienced drug or alcohol addiction during their lifetime.
- Approximately forty-six percent of that group had abused alcohol or were addicted to alcohol.
- About forty-one percent had abused drugs or were addicted to drugs.
- Alcohol is the most commonly abused substance among bipolar individuals.

Like substance abuse, BD poses a risk to the individual's physical and emotional well-being. Those afflicted with BD have a higher rate of relationship problems, economic instability, accidental injuries, and suicide than the general population. Such people are also significantly more likely to develop an addiction to drugs or alcohol.

SECOND EPISODE

CHAPTER FIVE SECOND EPISODE – PART 1 CALM BEFORE THE STORM

June 1998

It had been almost two years since the onset of my first bipolar episode. I was continuing on a strict regimen of medications and therapy sessions with my initial psychiatrist. It's difficult to say when one episode entirely ends and life returns to normal. I liken an episodic hospitalization to an earthquake that totally rattles your nerves for a relatively short time span. However, the future tremors or aftershocks, in some extreme cases, can continue for months or even years.

In retrospect, I may not have been properly medicated after my first episode. I had a constant stare, which may have signified overmedication. I was always drowsy. I trusted my doctor for his guidance and never questioned it. In fairness to the situation, there were multiple meds involved, sometimes referred to as cocktails. Without the proper dosages of each one, problems can ensue. At times, new drugs were substituted for existing ones. It was almost like a case of hit or miss since every person has a different chemical makeup.

Although I was obviously functional, and this was one of my milder episodes, I never felt entirely comfortable in the workforce under stress. I often had difficulty concentrating. I was a nervous wreck. I did take several vacations in a short timeframe around this period in which I was able to relax including my final trip to Australia in 1997. So there was some respite between the madness.

I was now working at a major software corporation leading up to the Y2K computer chaos. I reported to a sales manager for my first year as a sales support specialist. My manager Marc was the best boss I'd ever had. I struggled to be competent at times, but since I wasn't technical, I was like a penny waiting for change. What was I doing working at perhaps the most reputable software company in the nation? I could barely figure out how to log onto my laptop. Fortunately, I was a member of a five-person sales team, which helped pick up the slack.

I was invited and attended our corporate annual Gold Club sales award celebration in Munich, Germany. It was the second time in my life I had been recognized with such honors for exceptional performance. For reasons I can't explain, my ineptitude was also rewarded with an undeserved promotion.

My first year at the software firm I wound up making well into the six figures. Despite being somewhat overmatched with my technical handicap, it was one of only two times in fifteen years that I would clear this earnings hurdle.

July 1999

One of my roles in my new position as a field support representative was to help the salesforce market advanced services to large customers. These gold and silver packages included database administrators and onsite technicians, who were at a premium.

One day, management told me I needed to deliver a strategic sales presentation to our biggest client. Our account manager, Bryan, never liked me, and didn't want me aboard the team. He thought I wasn't product knowledgeable, so he went out of his way to make my life miserable.

I tried my best to perform well, despite the circumstances that unfolded during my second year with the company. This was around the time I had foolishly decided to discontinue my meds under the prodding of several influential people in my life, including my girlfriend, Charlene. Somewhat surprisingly, my psychiatrist gave me his blessing. I had learned through research that there are cases where patients with mental illness can function without medications, so ultimately it was my decision to give it a try.

My original doctor was the one responsible for my strict reliance on medication. To an extent, I had initially felt as though I was overmedicated, until he experimented with different drugs and dosages and discovered the correct combinations. Soon, I was beginning to feel somewhat better. It never dawned on me it was because I was now on the proper meds. It's difficult for me to establish an exact timeframe when this transpired since his office later burned down and all my medical records were destroyed.

It didn't help that the software company was easily the classiest organization, with the brightest people I had ever worked with. Everybody there was a veritable brain surgeon and, in my condition, I felt like I needed one. The worse my mental illness became, the more difficult it was for me to concentrate and control my racing thoughts.

Marcia and Martin, my director and manager, along with my supervisor Don, had me practice my presentation one hundred times until I had it down perfectly. I even took it home with me over the weekend.

Finally, the big day arrived.

Martin had a green SUV that he parked under the building in the parking garage. He told me that he and Don would wait for me while I followed them in my car. As luck would have it, an SUV like his pulled out of the driveway just before he did. I made the mistake of tailing it as it accelerated like a jackrabbit on steroids. I remember thinking to myself, why is he driving so fast if he knows I'm behind him?

I wound up trailing them until we reached Route 287 heading south. Even in my frazzled mind, I realized I should have been heading north. I turned around at the next exit to correct my mistake. It turns out I was only slightly off schedule since we had arranged to arrive early.

Naturally, Martin and Don gave me a hard time. "Where the hell were you?"

"I followed the wrong car," I replied sheepishly.

"What do ya mean, you followed the wrong car? What the hell's the matter with you?" There was considerable anger in Martin's voice.

I came close to telling them I have bipolar disorder and sometimes have trouble concentrating.

But Bryan was with us in the lobby as his customer contact came over to shake hands. Bryan was in his unprofessional glory.

"Hey, Frank," he said, "the guy giving your presentation today got lost coming here. He followed the wrong car. How funny is that?"

He was obviously trying to embarrass me, not realizing he was also ridiculing a company employee just before a major presentation worth over one million dollars. Not to mention he would be the one to benefit from it directly since it would be applied toward his sales quota. Fortunately, the customer ignored Bryan's immature comments, and we proceeded to the conference room. Marcia had now joined us, and the room was already filling up with ten or twelve client representatives.

After we set up the projector, the customer's director asked us to go around the room and introduce ourselves since there were a lot of new faces. Wouldn't you know it? When it was Bryan's turn, he froze and blurted out, "Hi, my name is B-b-b-b-b-ryan."

He stumbled over his own name. The guy got what he deserved. Thank you, God. By the way, the presentation went flawlessly. My practice had paid dividends.

***

Later That Month

After working at the software company for almost two years, I accepted a position at a much smaller communications provider, where my friend, Jonathan worked. It was late July 1999. I was hired as a sales engineer supporting the salesforce, which included Jonathan and four others. My manager was a gentleman named Glenn, who was one of my favorite bosses, albeit for only a short time.

I already had a two-week vacation to The Holy Land planned for August with my sister Linda, so my time off was approved. This trip would be the site of my second bipolar episode.

As mentioned, I was dating a Swiss woman at the time, Charlene. She was a pharmacist who wound up being a curse delivered by the Devil himself. Based on her version of the story that she conveyed in her French accent, I surmised that she had nagged her husband into becoming a heavy drinker. Apparently, this eventually led to his untimely death. She came home from work one day and discovered him sprawled out on their bed naked with an empty bottle of vodka in his hand. He was dead. She came very close to causing my demise as well.

We dated for only about three or four months, but she totally wreaked havoc on my life. She slept over my house one night and got out of bed before me the following fateful morning. She claimed to have accidentally discovered my medications while looking for a box of cereal. I had them buried behind cans and bottles on one of the shelves to ensure no one would find them. No one that is except Sherlock Charlene.

When I walked into the kitchen, I had no idea what was about to happen. She held up the bottles of my prescription drugs, and interrogated me, "How come you didn't tell me you were taking medications?"

I should have replied that it was none of her friggin' business.

Instead, I meekly purred, "Oh, them?" I motioned toward the bottles of pills she held in her outstretched hand.

"They're just to help me relax; I've been under a lot of stress lately," I said, forgetting she was a pharmacist, and would see through my lie.

"Liar. They're for bipolar disorder."

Once again, I should have stood up for myself and ordered her out of my house for prying into my personal stuff. After all, I had only known her for a short while.

"You don't need pills," she said. "You're fine. Promise me you won't take them anymore. You just need to exercise more and play tennis like you used to."

She was right about one thing. I was starting to look and feel fine, but it was because I was now finally on the correct meds. This is a mistake many mentally ill people in my position make, stopping their medications when they are working. I was also feeling pressured by an influential relative of mine, so I called my doctor and explained the situation. He reluctantly consented that I could safely give it a try short-term and, if things worsened, I could always resume taking them.

Famous last words . . .

CLINICAL OVERVIEW (CHAPTER FIVE)

*W*hat are some of the risks associated with discontinuing bipolar medications?

Pharmacological treatment is fundamental for successfully managing patients with bipolar disorder (BD). For acute episodes, the objective is symptom reduction, with the ultimate goal of full remission. For maintenance treatment, the goal is to prevent the recurrences of mood episodes. Medications used in the treatment of BD include mood stabilizers, atypical antipsychotics, and conventional antidepressants.

Medication nonadherence is a significant problem in primary care medicine in general, and in patients with BD in particular. It is probably the most important factor contributing to poor treatment outcome in BD.[18]

Most often, the first medicines used in addressing BD are mood stabilizers. They prevent mood swings and extreme changes in activity and energy levels. With proper medications, the patient may begin to feel better. In some instances, symptoms of mania may feel good, or side effects from the medications may occur. As a result, the patient may be tempted to cease taking them. However, stoppage of medicines, or improper change in dosages, can cause symptoms to return and worsen. If there are any questions or concerns, patients should consult with the provider[19].

The patient should call upon family members or friends to assist in the daily regimen to ascertain whether they are consuming the proper dosage of meds. This precaution can also guide them in ensuring that episodes of mania and depression are treated promptly. If mood stabilizers are not beneficial, the patient's provider may suggest other medicines, such as antipsychotics or antidepressants. The patient will require regular visits with a psychiatrist to discuss and monitor their medications and possible side effects. Blood tests are often needed, too.

In a study conducted in 2017, Dr. Laysha Ostrow and her colleagues surveyed two hundred and fifty mostly white and well-educated adults. They had been diagnosed with schizophrenia, psychosis, BD, or depression, and had tried to quit one or two medicines in the past five years. The survey population wasn't weighted to represent the demographics of the United States generally, so its respondents were heavily skewed. Still, Ostrow says, it provides insights into the experiences of many.

Among the survey results:

- The majority of respondents ceased their medicines with the support of their doctors, yet most didn't rate their doctors as helpful during the process.
- About three out of four respondents wanted to stop because of side effects.
- A little more than half of the survey-takers said they ran into severe withdrawal symptoms while quitting.[20]

CHAPTER SIX SECOND EPISODE – PART 2 HOLY LAND ADVENTURE

L inda and I left for Israel in August 1999. We wanted to visit before the millennium. I was already beginning to mentally downward spiral upon our arrival at the airport that hot and humid morning. I realized that I was losing my ability to concentrate as we awaited the remainder of our party to assemble near the baggage area. The guide, who was organizing our trip along with our fellow tourists, was waving a sign to identify the group. Fortunately, Linda was there to keep me from wandering in another direction.

On our drive from the airport to the hotel by van, I took in our entourage. There were two middle-aged Jewish women sitting alongside a black woman, whom we would later learn had a lifelong goal of being baptized in the Jordan River. There was an elderly married couple with the surname Kowalski, along with our guide.

I coughed excessively throughout the drive, which annoyed the other passengers, who were still recovering from jetlag. I would later discover this constant hacking to be a telltale sign of the onset of bipolar episodes.

***

The first night that we arrived in Amman, my sister and I consumed a late night snack in the hotel restaurant. During our conversation, she reminded me that I mentioned when we checked in at our initial hotel in Israel, I had climbed out of my window onto the ledge. I became worried when I had difficulty returning to my room from the window sill.

"You told me that you stopped taking your bipolar medication several weeks prior to our trip," she said.

She did not understand mental illness at the time, and later informed me she was very perplexed that I might be suicidal. She prayed for me and quoted scripture from Psalm 91:15-16: "He shall call upon me, and I will answer him: I will be with him in trouble; I will deliver him, and honour him. With long life will I satisfy him, and shew him my salvation." She wrote those verses on a piece of paper.

"Promise me that you'll meditate on them tonight."

Restless the next morning before dawn, I removed my shirt and sneakers, and went for a stroll in town. Before departing my hotel room, I placed the piece of paper with the verses Linda had given me on my pillow, and I left my door unlocked and slightly ajar. Her room was down the hallway, around the corner from mine.

I then walked shoeless past the back of our hotel and encountered a worker cleaning the pool. He paused and gazed at me as if I were contemplating diving into the water. Instead, I continued my barefoot journey into town. I met a food vendor setting up his wares for the day. I inquired in a raised whisper, "Do you have any food for me? I am poor and hungry."

He hastily motioned me away and shouted something in a mixed dialect about calling the police. I moved onward gingerly, with my bare feet blistering on the hot ground. In the distance, I spotted the Jordan River Hotel. Behind the hotel was a huge flowing body of water, which I deduced to be the Jordan River.

POLAR EXTREMES

As I approached the hotel, I noticed a large opening in the chain-link fence surrounding it. There were at least twenty people of various races and nationalities swimming in the water. I crawled through the hole and continued until I reached the water's edge. I soaked my tired feet. Then I waded into the river until I was submerged to my shoulders.

I said a prayer and lowered my head, baptizing myself as Jesus had. I had already been formally baptized at Times Square Church in New York City, but this experience in the Holy Land was much more spiritual.

My fellow travelers were in the hotel lobby having finished breakfast. Linda later told me that when I failed to join them, she hurried to my room searching for me. She observed that my door was slightly ajar. She opened it and discovered I had left my shoes and wallet behind. Then, she noticed the "long life" scripture she had written for me on my pillow, and she panicked. She alerted the tour guide that I was missing, and he involved the hotel personnel. One of the employees told my sister that a worker saw a barefoot man wearing only jeans and no shirt walking away from their hotel toward the Jordan River. The hotel security guard escorted Linda by car to see if they could spot me, but they were unsuccessful. The next stop for them was the Israeli Police Station.

Linda later assured me that the police officers were extremely nice to her. We had witnessed Israeli officers with machine guns at the airport, and they seemed intimidating. However, she said that, in person, the Israeli police were so kind and caring. After she explained to the police chief that I had been acting strangely the night before, and that I had left the "long life" scripture on my pillow case, he appeared worried.

"I'm concerned that he may have drowned in the Jordan River," she said.

The police chief was about to dispatch a helicopter crew to fly over the river to search for me. However, another officer entered the room and notified everyone that a woman had just called regarding my whereabouts.

The caller operated a local hostel, and she sighted me walking barefoot and shirtless on the road. She encouraged me to enter her car, and I was transported to her hostel. I vaguely recall her giving me a T-shirt provided by one of the youths staying there. The police officer relayed the address to the hotel security guard, and he drove Linda to meet me. When she saw me, she ran toward me, excited and relieved.

"Thank God that you're alive!"

I reacted indifferently to her display of emotions. "I didn't think that you would even come looking for me."

The woman from the hostel later explained to us that it was fairly common for first-time Israel visitors to have odd spiritual experiences like I did. Therefore, she was not overly concerned about assisting me when she saw me barefoot and shirtless on the street.

She said to me with a smile, "You are very lucky that your sister is such a Sherlock Holmes!"

I remember thinking that was a strange reference for someone to be making in Israel.

***

During our midsummer trip to Jerusalem, our mini-van tour group of seven passengers was led by a middle-aged, rotund, male guide with a mustache and dark complexion. He sported a Mickey Mouse T-shirt throughout most of our journey. One fellow sightseer was a strange, older, sinister man, with his wife, the Kowalski's I alluded to earlier. In my paranoid state of mind, I was convinced he was demonic because of his peculiar behavior and sensed he was continually staring at me and laughing.

I am a firm believer in the spiritual world. It was almost as if my bipolar episodes were drawing me into a new supernatural realm, as I embarked upon a mysterious trek on the dark side.

Mr. Kowalski constantly interrupted the guide throughout our trip, asking him to repeat himself. I suspected this was because he wore hearing aids and thick glasses, making it difficult for him to follow along. My mood swings flared and I had trouble controlling my temper. The scorching midday heat wasn't helping matters.

We had just arrived at the Garden Tomb, which was normally a tranquil setting of beautifully maintained trees and gardens. However, this sacred site where some Christians believe Jesus Christ was buried and resurrected, was in disarray. Scaffolding surrounded the entire rock structure, turning it into an eyesore. We were told the construction was necessary to prepare for the upcoming millennial celebrations beginning in January.

That didn't make sense to me. Shouldn't the sacred tomb be kept in its original state for posterity, not to mention tourists? Wasn't that the whole point? In my mind, I likened this to deciding to fix the ruins in Italy or Greece. And I thought I was crazy. We ran into this same situation throughout our travels in the Holy Land.

The city of Cana, where Jesus performed his first miracle by converting water into wine, was now a veritable junkyard infested with graffiti. Drawings and words spray-painted on the walls in a foreign language abounded. There were old, shredded rubber tires secured to the outside of the locked metal fence surrounding countless piles of garbage.

The serene area in the Jordan River where Jesus was baptized was undergoing massive reconstruction involving a large crane and noisy drilling. Bulldozers were tearing up the roads in Bethlehem, Christ's birthplace, and Nazareth. There was rubbish strewn everywhere in the vicinity of the Western Wall in Jerusalem. I remember wondering if it would be more appropriate to rename Israel the "Unholy Land." It seems as though the only grounds that were magnificently preserved were those exalting the pagan gods and goddesses.

It was now time to set foot in the Garden Tomb. The guide told us to remain quiet as we wandered inside. My sister and I followed Mr. Kowalski and his wife. Within seconds of entering the rock structure, Mr. Kowalski raised the volume of his voice to his wife.

"Be quiet," I said in a soft, but firm whisper.

He turned to face me with a confused look, and mumbled something.

"Shut up!" I said. Then I shoved him, making him stagger backwards, almost falling.

Linda stared in disbelief. "Why did you just push him?"

"Because, he was being irreverent; we're in the Garden Tomb."

"I can't believe you just did that! Are you feeling okay?"

"Yes, I'm fine." I half-smiled.

That was the last of our encounters with Mr. Kowalski. He and his wife steered clear of my sister and me for the remainder of our overall trip.

The following morning, we stopped the van out in the desert, near the place where Jesus had been tempted thrice by The Devil. I felt good that day. One of the interesting and fortunate aspects of bipolar disorder is the gaps between mania and depression. It's like these moments of relief are there to give your mind a respite before the next onslaught.

We brought our Bibles and took turns reading passages. During our spiritual journey throughout Israel, I was being consumed by an overwhelming desire to learn more about God. As I drifted from the group, I recalled a DVD I had watched just before our trip about the possibility of hidden messages in the original King James Version Bible. It usually applied to phrases that surfaced twice in proximity to each other and didn't appear together anywhere else within the sixty-six chapters.

As I stood there in solitude, I prayed silently. "God, reveal to me more about yourself. Please share with me something that I may know you better."

As if on cue, a sudden, gentle breeze swept across the desert and turned the pages of my open Bible to the "Song of Solomon." In Chapter One, verses five and six the following phrase was repeated.

"I *am* black, but comely . . ." and then again "Look not upon me, because I *am* black . . ."

Significantly, the word *am* in the book was already italicized.

My heartrate hastened. Had he revealed a message to me?

God, our Father, is black.

My brother, Tim, later told me this chapter pertained to King Solomon's concubine (mistress) who was black, and that these two quotes did not concern God himself. I understood Tim's explanation, but my contention was with the message itself. The desert breeze could have easily turned my open Bible to any of the remaining sixty-five chapters that day, but it didn't.

The Bible says that nobody has seen the face of God. Therefore, no one can disprove this claim with any certainty. And, what if it were true that He *is* black? Why would this fact be revealed to me, a white person? Perhaps because it would lend credibility to the discussion. Think about the impact it would have on a prejudiced world. Would it foster possible unity or further division among the masses? I found this to be an interesting thought with so many possibilities.

This revelation was one of several messages relayed to me by God during my bipolar episodes. I know most people would question my sanity regarding these so-called amazing discoveries. This was especially true since I was admittedly somewhat incoherent at the time. As a result, I told no one.

Another noteworthy point is that this curiosity only appears in the authentic original King James Version Bible. In the New King James Version, the word *black* is replaced with *dark.*

During our trip to Israel, we saw many tourist sites where dozens of people roamed, listening to oversized headset devices. This sight frightened me enormously. My paranoia had set in once again. I thought they were talking about me and attempting to read my mind. Linda assured me they were simply tourists like us who needed to have what they were viewing interpreted in their native languages.

I had mentioned earlier the black woman on our tour who had a lifelong desire to be baptized in the Jordan River. My sister and I decided to join her during that stop on our itinerary. I snapped photographs of the two of them baptizing each other, and it brought tears to my eyes.

Later in our trip, we arrived at perhaps my favorite stop, the Dead Sea. There were locker rooms for us to change into our swim trunks. I was having extreme difficulty focusing as throngs of men and boys were scurrying around me. My sister was in the women's locker room and in the chaos that ensued didn't notice I was missing from the group. They headed down the hill to the sea without me. I was sitting on a bench trying to concentrate. Suddenly, it dawned on me that I had been left behind. This was a once-in-a-lifetime attraction. I couldn't miss it. I had always wanted to float in the Dead Sea. If I had a bucket list, this would be high on it. The guide had announced earlier that this was a quick stop; we had only a half hour to enjoy it. The rest of the group had disappeared at least ten minutes ago.

There was only one choice. I had to somehow sprout wings and fly. The torn ligament in my left knee from my car accident six years before still impacted my mobility. While I sometimes wore a supportive brace when playing tennis and softball, under no circumstances should I run and risk further damage to the knee. However, the situation was dire, and I decided to perform my best impersonation of Tom Hanks in the movie, *Forrest Gump*, and made a mad dash down the hill.

I heard a feeble old lady cheering me from the side of the path as she pumped her tiny fist in the air. "Go get 'em, Tiger!"

Using Granny's battle cry as motivation, I threw my shoulders back and kept my arms and legs churning until I reached my destination. When I arrived, I was relieved to discover a portion of the group. I immediately jumped into the salt water and floated on my back. For someone who had never done the back float, let alone swim a day in his life, this was an amazing feat, and treat as well. I had somehow managed to set aside my bipolar condition for one fifteen-minute moment. I savored an experience I refused to let slip through my grasp.

Prior to dinner at our hotel that day, a DJ played the bizarre song "The Funky Chicken." This was presumably to enliven a bar mitzvah, or some happy hour celebration outside a nearby temple. For some reason, I pictured Jesus overturning the tables and throwing out the money lenders in anger, as he had in the Bible.

This out of place song reminded me of a melody that wouldn't escape my brain throughout our entire trip in the Holy Land. Since I write music, this wouldn't normally be unusual. During a two-month span, I had written nineteen new tunes. Because they were all compositions about God, I'm certain I was inspired by him to write them as worship and praise.

The song was titled "Baking." I interpreted its lyrics as a potential pun directed by God to the Devil: "You do the baking (in hell), and I'll do the making (creating)." My sister chastised me on several occasions for humming this melody too loudly, while riding on a

91

crowded elevator in our hotel. It had been composed by an acoustic guitar band duo from New Jersey that I had recently watched perform at a "first night" celebration in a neighboring town to mine back home.

The final part of our trip to Israel involved a rarity for Linda and me, flying home in the front row of first class. There was an electronic monitor on the wall facing us, tracking the flight back to New Jersey. The departure was delayed for about an hour because of a bomb scare. I watched the screen the entire way, frightened out of my paranoid wits that our plane would be shot down, and I would be the first to witness it.

December 1999 Back to Work

I began working at the small telecommunications company in July 1999, just prior to my excursion to the Holy Land. After my return, I drifted back and forth between normalcy and instability for the next several months. Soon it was Christmastime, and I suggested we all chip in for a gift for our manager, Glenn. When the idea was rejected by the group, I decided to buy him a separate present.

Later that week, senior management instructed us to refrain from purchasing any items for our bosses. Despite this announcement, Jonathan told me he had already ordered genuine Cuban cigars from an internet web site, which smuggled them into the country. He did this so he could one-up the rest of the sales group and buy Glenn a gift he would appreciate. Later, Jonathan boasted his desire for a new sales director promotion. Sure enough, he would wind up securing it.

There were many instances with Jonathan and Glenn where I was asked to go out for cocktails with the boss after work as a means of getting ahead.

Jonathan would continually chide me, "There are certainly worse things to do to advance your career than to go out drinking with the boss, even if you have other plans."

Glenn offered to promote me to sales director on at least two separate occasions—I'm still unsure if Jonathan was ever aware of those offers. I refused them since I was reluctant to participate in the corporate political good old boy network. As a humble and private person, I didn't want to create the mistaken impression that I was receiving something that wasn't based entirely on merit. The additional money simply wasn't worth it to me.

I wound up working at this place for eight months culminating in mid-March 2000. What had started out as my favorite job of my career, had taken a major detour. It was here I experienced the pinnacle of my second bipolar episode.

It was around this time that I informed Jonathan about my most recent girlfriend's permanent departure from my life. Her name was Cindy, and he had met her at our office Christmas party. Predictably, he wisecracked, "You're better off. She was white trash, trailer park anyway."

He attributed this statement to the fact she drank Zinfandel at the party. Jonathan wasn't the most sensitive guy in the world.

There was another incident where he criticized my Christian beliefs, and admitted he used a Ouija Board, which I found to be offensive. He boasted about the time he inquired of it as to how far he would advance in his career. He said it responded: "director." When he asked it the first name of the person who would promote him, it replied. "Karl." Both predictions would ultimately come true. Spooky.

The Millennium – January 2000

As an unpublished songwriter, I was now visiting the studio nightly to record the significant number of songs I had written while in the Holy Land. I had foolishly followed the advice of my ex-girlfriend Charlene and my doctor, and had stopped taking my meds. I was destined for a fall. Along with the rigors associated with my new job, problems ensued.

My job and recording studio performances began to rapidly deteriorate, both physically and mentally, due to sleep deprivation and long, stressful hours. I was exhausted. I was in the throes of determining whether I should bother continuing to pursue a love life at all. As I sat in the office one day, my eyes focused on an object of sentimental value.

It was a romantic photograph of me and Cindy, taken at a fine restaurant. As was the case with Charlene, who I had dated earlier, Cindy had broken up with me after a short-term relationship. This split was also a result of my reluctant divulging to her of my deep, dark secret: that I had bipolar disorder. I had unwisely told her too much, including my fleeting thoughts of suicide. She hurried out of my house, shouting hurtful words to the effect of me posing a potential threat to cause her bodily harm because of my unstable condition.

In fairness to Cindy, she probably felt guilty after spewing those childish remarks. This became evident when she telephoned me the following week with a dinner invitation to her home in Pennsylvania.

Her two teenaged daughters, who I hadn't yet met, were at the dinner. Cindy even cooked one of my favorite meals, veal cutlet parmesan over linguini, and a salad.

Her daughters took one look at me towering in their doorway, and it was hate at first sight. They cast dirty looks at me and didn't invite me to come in. Cindy had warned me in advance that they missed their father dearly since her recent divorce, and not to take their rudeness personally. I knew I was in trouble at dinner when I politely asked one of them to please pass me the salad dressing, and she refused. This was despite her mother's insistence. I told myself my chances of a reconciliation at this stage with this woman are slim.

Later in January 2000

When my colleagues and I were in Atlanta at our Sales Kickoff Meeting in January, I had separated from the New Jersey group and was chatting with a fellow Christian named Dana. She was visiting from another office. We were discussing God and our spiritual beliefs. Deliberately mistaking our intent, the New Jersey sales contingency began mocking me when she went to the ladies room.

"So, Steve, are you going to bang her?" shouted one of the drunken fools.

"Yeah, West, when are you going to do her?" laughed another idiot.

"So, when are you going to close the deal?" chimed in yet another one.

Obviously, I viewed these comments as infantile, but I knew these guys were immature and inebriated. Because of this, Dana and I chose to leave the party separately. Before she did, she made disparaging remarks to me about the poor quality of sales people in the New Jersey office. I shook my head in disgust when they followed us into the lobby to see if we entered the elevator together.

Arnie, one of our sales reps, had become verbally abusive to me in front of Dana. In his stupor, he referred to me as a *stringy mutant gnome*, whatever that meant. The guy was really strange, to say the least.

Later that night, I was sprawled on my hotel room floor in a manic state, unable to sleep. I was writing hysterical gibberish about Arnie, which somehow made sense to me in the moment. I wish I still had those writings.

I found out the following morning that Arnie had supposedly swung an empty wine bottle at our eastern region vice-president. I'm not sure if he missed or not, but amazingly he wasn't fired.

On our way home from Atlanta, I sat in an airport lounge with Jonathan, along with our sales rep Greg and Alan, a high-level executive. Alan innocently offered to buy us a round of drinks. Greg had confided in me on a prior occasion he was a recovering alcoholic. I was a former problem drinker, having been on an employee assistance program back in 1993, so liquor was out of the question. Of course there was no way for Alan to know any of this.

Jonathan knew about our drinking situations. When Greg and I ordered a Coke, Alan initially poked fun at us. "What's the matter? Don't you guys drink?"

Greg and I politely objected to his persistent prodding. "No, thank you, but I appreciate the offer," we responded almost in unison. This would be the first of many times I had to turn down alcohol because of my fear of it clashing with my bipolar condition. Alan smiled diplomatically and withdrew his offer.

Later, Jonathan, the troublemaker, would reprimand me for exercising poor judgment. Once again, I had turned down a gesture from a high-ranking executive. This could have helped advance my career from a politically correct standpoint into the good old boy network. When would I ever learn?

Mid–February 2000

Shortly after the trip, I returned to the recording studio. I had coordinated with Dan, the studio owner and producer who was blind, and Jack, the arranger, to hire three twelve-year-old girls to provide the lead vocals on four of my new Christian songs. They were very professional and had experience performing for a local choir. After they recorded the melodies, Dan tripled their vocals to create the auditory illusion of a full choir. I was ecstatic with the results.

One of the mothers accompanied them to the studio that afternoon. Because one of my songs openly opposed abortion, it presented a sensitive topic to pro-choice listeners. Dan expressed some initial concern that the trio would back out. Fortunately, this was not the case.

I had developed a nasty sinus infection earlier in the week. This was unusual for me, since I almost never got physically sick . . . my mental illness was sufficient. The bottle of pills the clinic gave me contained hundreds of miniscule yellow tablets. For some reason, I had the notion they were sleeping pills.

I don't recall being particularly depressed, but mood swings are funny. I casually decided to overdose on the pills. I was standing at my kitchen counter, removing the cap from the bottle. I tilted my head back and emptied the entire bottle into my mouth. I coughed up many of them, and they scattered across the room. I grasped the tiny container, tossed it into the sink, and proceeded to lie down on the tiled floor. I figured I would painlessly die in my sleep.

I lived on an exceptionally quiet cul-de-sac, a few doors from the end of the block. There was typically complete stillness outside, and this Saturday morning was no different. I didn't even hear birds chirping. Lying motionless on the kitchen floor, I felt certain I had died and the world had stopped turning.

Eventually, I heard a car roll slowly by. This barely audible sound was enough to wake me from my light slumber. I propped myself up and stared at the wall clock. It was a few minutes before one. My studio session was scheduled to begin momentarily. I was incredibly dizzy. My hands shook uncontrollably. My nerves were further rattled by the loud, sudden ringing of the telephone. It was Dan.

"Where the hell are ya?"

I was typically fifteen minutes early to the studio. Obviously, today would be different. This Saturday was especially poor timing on my part since Dan didn't open the studio on weekend afternoons. He was doing me a favor to accommodate my schedule. Besides, the three girls were coming to sing. It was totally inconsiderate on my part.

"I'm so sorry; I lost track of time."

"What do ya mean you lost track of the time?" He was understandably livid. "The girls are already here. We're gonna have to start without you!"

"I'm on my way. I'll be there in half an hour."

Adrenaline gave me a new burst of energy. I hustled out the door. Normally, it took me forty-five minutes to make it to the studio, but true to my word, I was scurrying up the stairs into the second-floor loft in exactly thirty minutes. The session was already in full swing. Fortunately, I had laid down the reference vocals to the songs earlier in the week, so the girls were able to practice the melodies while they waited for me.

Dan was still furious with me for being late. Thankfully, since he was blind he couldn't see my hands tremoring like crazy from devouring the pills. This would have made him even more curious as to the cause for my lateness. The session was flawless. Amazingly, the girls performed the four songs on one take! This is an outstanding accomplishment even for seasoned adult vocalists but they were experienced choir singers.

As the session ended and Dan confirmed the vocals were perfect, the girls donned their coats and headed toward the exit. They looked like three young geese following each other in single file. I had made arrangements with their mothers to pay them for their efforts. However, they apparently hadn't been told about the payment and thought they were performing for free. This was probably because they didn't get paid for the choir work, but I wanted to pay them for their talent and hard work on my songs.

"No, wait, come back!" I shouted.

Surprised, they turned and headed back. I asked their names as I wrote out a one hundred and fifty dollar check for each of them. Their faces broke into wide smiles, which made me feel happy.

"Oh, goodie, now I can buy some new clothes at the mall!" said one of the girls.

When they went their way, I thought, "All's well that ends well." But my euphoria was short-lived. Dan began chastising me again for being late, and for my overall strange behavior. His sound engineer had told him about my hand shaking when I was writing out the checks.

As I navigated my way to the door, I spotted the large plastic bone Dan kept for his seeing-eye dog on the floor. When the sound engineer turned his back, I scooped it up and hid it in the pocket of my jacket. I said my goodbyes and headed downstairs and out of the building. There was a mailbox on the corner. As I strolled by, I pulled back the lid, and deposited the bone inside for no reason, other than a personal chuckle. I would have loved to have seen the look on that mailman's face.

In fairness to Dan, I had been acting strange lately. One night I inexplicably raced into the studio, carrying the insert cover to one of my cassettes: *Boy from Jersey*. I had Dan convinced by my insistence that there were evil spirits out to get him and he needed to carry this good luck charm to ward them off. I could tell by his horrified expression that he was scared out of his wits, and who could blame him? The most peculiar thing of all was he somehow still believed me.

In a frenzy, I begged him to grab one of my reel-to-reel tapes and have his sound engineer play it backwards on his equipment. I insisted it contained a hidden, cryptic message, similar to *The Beatles'* song claiming "Paul is dead." To my astonishment, I had him once again so spooked he thought I might be right. In retrospect, I was experiencing a severe paranoid stage of my lingering episode. When they played the tape backwards, there was nothing but garbled sound, no hidden message, nothing. I now had lost all credibility with Dan, and deservingly so.

***

Of the four tunes, I was particularly pleased with the final production of "Song for Jesus." It had a two-part instrumental featuring a string section that created an orchestral effect. It was catchy. I drove around town for hours one afternoon with a demo copy of the cassette blaring in my car stereo. I began finger-tapping the steering wheel in rhythm, trying to act cool like Richard Gere in *American Gigolo.* I pulled into a gas station and rolled down the window.

"Hey, boss, what'll it be?" asked the attendant.

I was bopping to the music. "Fill it up, regular . . . I'm Richard Gere."

The guy second-glanced at me and rolled his eyes. It's like I could read his mind. He was thinking: another nut case.

On the way home, I picked up the Sports Illustrated Swimsuit Edition that is published each February. As expected, there was a beautiful model on the cover. I envisioned she was my girlfriend, Cindy, whom I had stopped seeing after our brief fling. I showed off my artistic flair by drawing a valentine around her navel with her name and mine engraved in ink.

Physically enticed by the beautiful poses of the models, I paged meticulously through the magazine. Sitting down at my dining room table, I penned a love letter to Cindy. I vaguely remember blaming my strange behavior on my bipolar condition, telling her I loved her and pleading with her to take me back.

When my sister Linda visited me for dinner, I showed her the letter. "So, what do you think?"

She scanned it, as her face lit up in horror. "You're not going to send this to her, are you?"

"Yeah, why, what's the problem?"

"You can't tell her you love her! You'll scare her away for good. You were only dating for a few months."

She tossed the letter back on the table and stormed out of the room. "Do what you want, but I think you're crazy."

"You're right. I am crazy; that's the problem."

"Just say a prayer tonight and God will guide you with his wisdom," she said.

I slept on it that night, and in the morning decided my sister was right. I tore the pages to shreds.

I did call Cindy one final time in an attempt for closure of our failed relationship. It was very awkward. I asked her if she had held onto the gold angel pin that I bought her when we first met. She collected angels.

"Yes, of course, but it's Cupid."

"I'm not sure what you mean."

"The pin. It's not an angel . . . it's Cupid."

"Oh? Is that good?"

"Well, I don't know. It is for Valentine's Day, I suppose."

We shared a final chuckle, then hung up and went on with our separate lives.

CLINICAL OVERVIEW (CHAPTER SIX)

W*hat are the effects of religious/spiritual beliefs on the treatment of bipolar disorder and other mental illnesses?*
Research suggests that religious belief can help lessen symptoms of depression, but a study at Rush University Medical Center goes one step further.

In patients diagnosed with clinical depression, belief in a concerned God can improve response to medical treatment, according to a paper in the Journal of Clinical Psychology[21].

A total of one hundred and thirty-six adults diagnosed with major depression or bipolar disorder at inpatient and outpatient psychiatric care facilities in Chicago participated in the study. The patients were surveyed shortly after admission for treatment, and then again eight weeks later, each time using the Beck Depression Inventory, the Beck Hopelessness Scale, and the Religious Well-Being Scale – all standard instruments for assessing intensity, severity, depth of disease, feelings of hopelessness, and spiritual satisfaction.

Positive response to medication, defined as a fifty percent reduction in symptoms, can vary in psychiatric patients. Some may not respond at all. But the study found that those with strong beliefs in God were more likely to experience an improvement. Specifically, participants with clinical depression who scored in the top third of the Religious Well-Being Scale were seventy-five percent more likely to get better with medical treatment.

The researchers tested whether the explanation for the improved response was linked to the feeling of hope, which is typically a feature of religious belief. But degree of hopefulness, measured by feelings and expectations for the future and degree of motivation, did not predict whether a patient fared better on anti-depressants.

"In our study, the positive response to medication had little to do with the feeling of hope that typically accompanies spiritual belief," said Patricia Murphy, PhD, a chaplain at Rush and an assistant professor of religion, health and human values at Rush University. "It was tied specifically to the belief that a Supreme Being cared."

"For people diagnosed with clinical depression, medication certainly plays an important role in reducing symptoms," Murphy said. "But when treating persons diagnosed with depression, clinicians need to be aware of the role of religion in their patients' lives. It is an important resource in planning their care."

George Fitchett, PhD, also a chaplain at Rush and the director of the religion, health and human values program at Rush University, co-authored the study.

A separate source purports that religious and spiritual factors are increasingly being examined in psychiatric research. Religious beliefs and practices have long been linked to hysteria, neurosis, and psychotic delusions. However, recent studies have identified another side of religion that may serve as a psychological and social resource for coping with stress.

After defining the terms religion and spirituality, this paper reviews research on the relation between religion and (or) spirituality, and mental health, focusing on depression, suicide, anxiety, psychosis, and substance abuse. The results of an earlier systematic review are discussed, and more recent studies in the United States, Canada, Europe, and other countries are described. While religious beliefs and practices can represent powerful sources of comfort, hope, and meaning, they are often intricately entangled with neurotic and psychotic disorders, sometimes making it difficult to determine whether they are a resource or a liability[22].

CHAPTER SEVEN
SECOND EPISODE –
PART 3 AT THE OFFICE

In March of 2000, I accompanied Arnie on a sales call to his former office of employment. He exhibited extremely poor salesmanship during our visit. They had recently signed a one-year term agreement, and Arnie was advising them to make decisions that were not in their best interest. As he spoke, I was drifting in and out of coherency, losing the battle with reality.

The client repeatedly left the room, probably because of the unprofessional bickering between Arnie and me. I berated him several times during the customer's absence to concentrate our efforts on the replacement of existing basic telephone lines. He refused to listen. We left without the sale.

As we departed dejectedly, I was distracted by a curious abstract painting on the far wall of the conference room. Upon closer study, it reminded me of a pygmy engaging in a headhunting expedition in New Guinea. In my bipolar state of mind, he resembled a diminutive Arnie. I briefly contemplated snatching the painting and scurrying to the parking lot. I sometimes wonder whether I would have successfully confiscated it had I been so bold.

My condition was worsening. Concentration was difficult, especially at work. Whenever I attempted to form an intelligent thought, somebody would rudely interrupt me. This was particularly true for our sales rep, Kevin. I once confided my spiritual beliefs to him, in an attempt to motivate him into reading the Bible. When we returned to the office, he mocked me as he relayed our conversation to the rest of the group.

Then there was Sam. He exercised incredibly foolish judgment by practically dragging me to a customer site to help close a deal. I was so zoned out that day, he had to carry my briefcase and place it in my outstretched hand. After we registered with security, we headed to meet our contact. When I extended my hand for our customary handshake, I missed! Stumbling, I came close to toppling over. The customer immediately sensed something was awry and snarled, first at Sam and then in my direction.

Sam cleared his throat. "Steve is our sales engineer whom we have assigned to support your project. He is an expert concerning voice and data." Sam gestured to me as the fuming customer waited for my response.

Trying my hardest to act professionally, I chose to remain silent. I knew from previous experience that I would ramble if I opened my mouth. At one inappropriate time, Sam suddenly began chortling out loud. The client wasn't amused. Neither was I. Fortunately, the call passed quickly although we didn't get the sale. This would wind up being my penultimate day at the company. Thanks, Sam.

As I left the building that evening, I paused for the elevator on the top floor of our office. One of our sales reps, Bob, waited with me. He began to chuckle as I stood patiently. Dazed and confused once again, I had watched the lift repeatedly ascend and descend to and from our level, as I remained there motionlessly. Eventually, he had to guide me out of the building, or I might still be standing there.

Causing Chaos

For lack of a better word, my last day at work was surreal. I had to convince myself at times it was really happening. One of the sales people in our out-of-state office, Michele, needed my assistance in pricing a high-speed circuit. It was a rush, and their sales engineer was out sick that day. Normally, this request would have been a simple exercise. I could cost these circuits in my sleep. But now I couldn't concentrate. I was almost near the end of my downward spiral, ready to crash.

My inability to help Michele would be the trigger for my termination. I still can't believe what happened, but there are witnesses who swear to it. Apparently I downloaded an intimate photograph of Cindy and me from our office Christmas party. I attached it to an email and sent it to my entire distribution list, including many of our customers! My telephone suddenly began ringing wildly from fellow coworkers and clients notifying me of my mistake, so I realized it must be true.

Arnie, who occupied the cubicle next to mine, shouted over our shared wall, "You stupid son of a bitch!"

My mood swings were in full flow. I was a firecracker ready to explode. We jawed back and forth. Finally, I shouted, "Arnie, shut up, or I'm gonna fucking kill ya!"

I remember stalking the office after that. One of the reps was cowering at his desk. I stormed over to our boss, Glenn's secretary. "Please call Glenn and ask him to come to the office right away. It's very important."

As if she didn't already know that. I had been screaming bloody manslaughter, and threatening a fellow employee. I plopped calmly down across from Glenn's desk awaiting his arrival.

When he returned shortly thereafter from a site visit, he strode into his office where I was slumped in a chair and almost in shock. That wasn't me who had made those death threats . . . except it *was* me. Once again, I had experienced the horrors of bipolar disorder.

Glenn closed the door and sat down staring at me. "What the hell just happened?"

I wasn't in the mood to talk, so I avoided his inquisition. "Glenn, I think it's best if I resign, and we just leave it at that." I slid a barely legible, hand-scrawled letter across his desk.

Then I noticed his left hand was trembling, and it reminded me of something Jonathan, the instigator, had once mentioned, "Did you ever notice Glenn's left hand shakes?"

Truthfully, I hadn't until Jonathan had pointed it out to me. But now when I reiterated Jonathan's cruel comment to Glenn in our closed-door meeting, he countered, somewhat out of character, "Jonathan told me you're neurotic."

I ignored this stinging remark and repeated my earlier intention to simply resign.

"Why don't you go home tonight and think it over. We can talk about it again in the morning, okay?" He sounded kind and compassionate to my situation. We had always gotten along well, with mutual respect.

I reluctantly agreed. As I made my way to the door, the rest of the office was so quiet you could practically hear their hearts pounding. Surprisingly, nobody had called the police.

I resigned my position as sales engineer on March 8, 2000. Glenn originally told me to take some time to reconsider. However, our corporate executives apparently told him to move forward with a dismissal, rather than waiting for my termination. On the very next day, I received a termination letter from him with the following verbiage:

Dear Steve,

During our conversation Wednesday afternoon, you were very adamant about resigning from the company effective immediately. You went so far as to provide me with a written resignation letter. I had indicated that I would hold the resignation until Monday, March 13. I have given additional thought to our discussions. I do not think there is any benefit to providing you with additional time to reconsider your actions. Since you have already provided me with your company equipment, I will be processing your resignation effective March 10, 2000. You will receive your final paycheck next Friday and it will include pay through this date along with pay for your unused paid time off. Your employee benefits will end on March 31, 2000 and information regarding continuation of benefits will be sent to your home in the next two weeks.

Sincerely,

Glenn

There was one other funny, manic anecdote that took place the day I resigned, just before I exploded at Arnie. Our back-to-back cubicles in the corner of the office faced the door leading to the hall. Whenever a coworker would temporarily leave the area, they would pass us on the way out and upon their return. This usually happened with little warning because of our proximity to the exit.

I gazed up at the wall adjacent to the doorway, just out of sight of Arnie's view and began hallucinating. Hillary Clinton's face was projecting on the wall, and she was making funny faces at me. I giggled uncontrollably as she moved her lips.

Employees continued to exit and reenter through the door. As they did, I struggled to muffle my laughter. I prayed no one would pass my cubicle and discover my delirious state. Fortunately, I escaped embarrassment. Thirty minutes later, I was threatening to kill a coworker . . . talk about sudden mood swings.

***

At the Recording Studio

During my final week at the telecommunications company, I was attempting to lay down reference vocals to a composition I had written. These were needed for the studio singer who would be performing the actual final rendition of the song. They needed to have a clear understanding of my desired melody and lyrics. This one was titled, "Whatever." It was separate from the tunes I had recently recorded with the young girl vocalists. I had written or co-written all my music, so I should have known every lyric, verse, chorus and bridge. Unfortunately, this was no longer the case.

I was having an incredibly nerve-racking time trying to decide when to sing the final verse of the song. Since it was comprised of shorter than average lyrics, my arranger had compensated by extending the instrumental piece. I kept either entering too soon or waiting too long and missing my spot. Sometimes in situations like this, there was an expression Jack and I would say, "Count me in." He would stand on the other side of the glass and motion with his fingers: one . . . two . . . three . . . four. I was supposed to come in on the second "one."

I missed my cue at least six or seven times. I kept pleading with him. "Jack, count me in."

I was in mental anguish because I couldn't concentrate in my unstable condition. Tears welled up in my eyes as I begged him, "Jack, count me in." He remained patient. Every time the troublesome part came around, he would motion with his fingers for me again.

It seemed like an eternity in hell. And then it dawned on me. The lyrics to the song I was stumbling in agony over were, "Eternity will last forever. . ."

POLAR EXTREMES

It gave me something to think about on my drive home that night.

***

I have been an amateur songwriter since 1983 when I penned my first of one hundred and thirty songs. Over the following thirty-year period, I proceeded to create and record four or five new ones every year. Amazingly, during the two-month span surrounding my trip to Israel, I composed nineteen new Christian works. Something, or someone, had deeply inspired me. The answer was apparent to me.

My initial music from the eighties had included lyrics such as: "Where are all the Blondes?" and "Shakespeare Never Worked in ShopRite." The latter commemorated my supermarket days working during a union strike while putting myself through college.

This supermarket picket line that I'm in
Is a tangled web I'm doing time in.
In my head, old Shakespeare's words are rhymin',
And what to be or not to be is now the question facing me . . .
But, Shakespeare never worked in ShopRite – if he did, he'd know
It's so hard to do your job right; there's no place to go.
Staring out into the twilight, feeling mighty low.
Shakespeare never worked in ShopRite – if he did, he'd know. . .

When I returned from the Holy Land, I immediately made my way to the studio to record my nineteen new songs. These numbers were much more meaningful to me than the ones from my earlier days since they were a reflection of my newfound spirituality. I had them only in my head until that point, and my mind was drifting between reality and fantasy. I hired two female singers as alternating vocalists on the

111

majority of the pieces. Halfway through the sessions, one of them stated the obvious. "Gee, Steve, it looks like someone has become very religious recently," she said, smiling and sweetly.

I just grinned as she continued to knock out tune after tune on the first take, the mark of a true professional.

The average cost of a song recorded on 24-track reel-to-reel, which was the state-of-the-art technology before the advent of computers in the studio, was one thousand dollars. That meant the overall expense to record this compact disc was almost twenty thousand dollars. Fortunately, I was employed at the major software corporation in the highest paying job of my career, so I was able to afford it. Between my penchant for world travel and songwriting, I had two of the most expensive hobbies imaginable.

***

A few days before my next studio session, Jack had visited my house as he always did to review my new songs. He lugged his portable keyboard up the stairs of my townhouse, gasping for air. This constant struggle was the result of too little exercise and too many Pall Malls. To save money, he and I would rehearse the melodies before recording in the studio.

That night when Jack arrived, my place was in disarray. My clothes were flung over chairs, the dining room table, or crumpled in balls on the floor. I hadn't shaved or showered in days. This is a telltale signal of a bipolar disorder episode: not caring about your appearance, hygiene or personal surroundings. We had to step carefully around the scattered clothes and empty food containers to find a place to set up his equipment.

Jack pretended not to notice any of these out-of-character signs. He continued as if it were business as usual, even though I clearly sensed he noticed my strange behavior. I vividly recall one of the songs we finished recording that night since it contained the only instrumental I have ever co-written. At one point, my eyes filled with tears. I'm not sure why. Maybe it was because I felt the lyrics were so touching. Maybe I was finally realizing after all these years that Jack was in it just for the money.

Many of the song titles of my new Christian music were taken straight from the Bible, such as "Well Done, Faithful Servant," "Come, Follow Me," and "Suffer the Little Children." Some of the lyrics to my melodies were also based on quotes from scripture, such as Matthew 6:20-21: "Lay up for yourselves treasures in heaven, where thieves do not break in and steal. For where your treasure is, there your heart be also," and Matthew 7:7: "Ask, and it will be given you; seek, and you will find."

Last Day at Work

On the night of March 8, 2000, I left my job at the telecommunications company for the last time. I headed to the studio for my nocturnal recording session. I had an impossible time remembering how to leave the city. As always, my car was parked in the lot across from the office building. I was so confused, I drove around the block five times. When I finally arrived safely at the studio, I was late, which was highly unusual. I hustled upstairs to the second floor.

The tracks were already laid down on several of the tunes, and now it was my turn to deliver the reference vocals. I was able to complete the first song from start to finish without a hitch. Then I felt that old familiar feeling. I was getting ready to crash and I became extremely agitated. Although I made a valiant effort, I was unable to control myself or to concentrate. My knees were starting to buckle. The room was beginning to spin.

The title was "Everybody Loves Raymond, but Nobody Loves Jesus." I changed the chorus in the song and replaced *Raymond* with a friend from work's surname preceded by an expletive. The three people in the studio at that time were the owner and producer, who was blind, the arranger, and the sound engineer.

My memory temporarily blacked out at this juncture, but apparently I was ranting and raving at the studio owner who chastised me for messing up the lyrics to the song. "Dan, I'm gonna fucking kill ya!" Does this threat sound familiar? Once again, my bipolar condition had exposed homicidal thoughts, this time to a friend.

At this point, I was bleary-eyed as I tried to focus on Jack, who was storming angrily towards me. I leaned against an elevated stool I had been sitting on while performing the reference vocals, certain I was about to devour a knuckle sandwich. Instead he just towered over me. Eventually, I was able to stand up and stagger out of the studio's sound-proof area. Jack followed close behind, ensuring I wouldn't go near his blind, defenseless friend Dan who remained seated at the mixing board.

The bizarre ending to this event is that the sound engineer, caught up in the mayhem that ensued, had accidentally left the soundtrack tape running. Days later, Dan scheduled a female vocalist into the studio to rehearse a song. As he was locating the tracks for that tune, he accidentally raised the levels on the one where I had gone ballistic. He quickly lowered the sound level, but not before the vocalist gasped, "Oh, my God. Who was that yelling?"

Dan was quick to respond by changing the subject and distracting her. The scary part was how close I'd come to revealing the serious nature of my bipolar disorder illness.

CLINICAL OVERVIEW (CHAPTER SEVEN)

W *hat is homicidal ideation and its link to bipolar disorder and other mental illnesses?*
Homicidal ideation is a common medical term for thoughts about homicide. It defines the range of homicidal thoughts, which stretches from vague ideas of revenge to detailed and fully formulated plans without the act itself. Most people who have homicidal ideation do not commit homicide. However, seventy-six percent of five hundred and fifty-six random women, age twenty, and ninety-one percent of six hundred and twelve random men, age twenty, who participated in a research study in a Central Texas community, admitted to having had a homicidal fantasy[23]. Homicidal ideation is common, accounting for ten to seventeen percent of patient admissions to psychiatric facilities in the United States[24].

Serious thoughts about killing another person suggest a lack of coping skills. These ideas usually indicate psychological distress. Drug-induced delirium and psychosis are the most common conditions linked to homicidal ideation. Psychosis accounts for eighty-nine percent of hospital admissions associated with homicidal ideation in the United States[25]. Psychosis can also be drug-induced or related to other illnesses such as schizophrenia. Personality disorders such as borderline personality disorder, paranoid personality disorder, or antisocial personality disorder have also been known to cause thoughts of homicide.

Persons with acute mania can present in either inpatient or outpatient settings. Patients with a previous diagnosis of bipolar disorder may display severe manic episodes, defined by suicidal ideation, homicidal ideation, psychosis, or aggression.

Available data supports that homicide is overwhelmingly perpetrated by men compared to women. A review was undertaken involving current literature on men's mental health with a focus on assessing and reducing homicide risk in men with psychiatric conditions.

The results imply that bipolar disorder and schizophrenia share a biological trait that is a risk factor for homicide. Dual disorders, or the presence of a substance use disorder with other major mental illness, are a major risk factor for homicide in males. Dual diagnosis disorders, personality disorders and pathological traits and male depression share emotion dysregulation, irritability, and reactive aggression. Promoting physician education and addressing firearm safety are recommended. Other proposed measures include reducing the reluctance of men relative to women to engage in help-seeking behavior and using targeted risk interviews that integrate these data.

In conclusion, the main focus in prevention of homicidal behavior in males with psychiatric disorders should be to identify high risk groups, and to provide adequate treatment. It is also wise to facilitate compliance with long-term therapy while considering male specific problems and needs.

CHAPTER EIGHT SECOND EPISODE – PART 4 LATER THAT NIGHT

March 2000

After my behavior at the recording studio Dan knew something was obviously wrong. He was unfamiliar with the term bipolar disorder. He thought I had simply gone crazy overnight. After threatening him, I had headed in his direction with Jack shadowing me. Suddenly, I performed a back flop onto the couch in front of the mixing board. I started singing silly lyrics to familiar melodies. "On top of old Smokie I'll spend all my life, on top of old Smokie 'cause Smokie's my wife."

"Steve, you're gonna lose your job," he said, unaware I had just resigned.

"Relax, I'm just having some fun."

It was the end of the session, and the studio was ready to close. Dan's friend, Mitch, who was also blind, dropped by and sat down in the waiting room. He had a seeing-eye dog, too. The sound engineer was shutting down the equipment for the night.

Dan turned to Jack and pleaded, "Why don't you take Steve home? He's in no condition to drive."

"I don't want to get involved." Jack said, sounding annoyed.

I don't want to get involved! I echoed Jack's words in my head. What a jerk. After the tens of thousands of dollars I had lined his pockets with over the years, and now the guy wouldn't even give me a ride home. In my condition, I could have easily died that night. I guess you find out who your friends are in a crisis.

I had paid Dan more than seventy thousand dollars for his services. He was a professional and the songs were always recorded to my liking. On the other hand, Jack often showed up unprepared.

***

Now Mitch was playfully hollering to me from the waiting room. "Why don't you ask Dan to take you home?"

So I obliged: "Can you drive me home tonight?"

Mitch chuckled loudly from across the hall, "Steve, he's blind!"

Dan and Mitch shared a laugh at my expense.

"That's okay, guys, I can make it home on my own."

"Are you sure you're okay?" asked Dan.

"It doesn't look like I have much choice."

Jack had already left.

"We'll check on you in the morning to make sure you made it home safely," Mitch promised.

I said goodbye and headed out the door. I would be lying if I told you I remembered how I drove home that night. My car was on autopilot. Once again, my guardian angel must have been watching over me.

I do remember the violent wind gusts that night. On the back deck of my wooden townhouse branches rustled, and the wind chimes swayed like crazy. I was certain there was somebody trying to break into my house through the sliding glass door. So what did I do? Naturally, I called 9-1-1.

The police showed up promptly, and I apparently convinced them about the prowler. We headed around back; they shone their flashlights around my deck searching for footprints. Finding none, they assured me everything was fine, and I was pacified enough to go to bed. I was certain I saw one of them glance at his partner and roll his eyes as they left.

***

Mitch called me the following morning. Dan must have given him my telephone number.

I started shouting into the phone. "I need help! I'm losing it!"

"Give me your address, so I can call the cops," Mitch replied, trying to sound calm.

He told me he was summoning the police, and to unlock the front door so they wouldn't have to break in. Mitch helped save my life that day. After our call, I put on a pair of gym shorts and stumbled down the stairs into my living room. I sprawled out on the couch with a view of the sliding glass door leading out onto the back deck.

Minutes later, there was loud pounding on my front door. The police. It suddenly dawned on me I hadn't heeded Mitch's advice to unlock it. It also occurred to me that this was the second call to 9-1-1 made to dispatch the police to my residence in a matter of hours.

I made a valiant attempt to lift myself off the couch, to no avail. Fortunately, the two officers circled around back, peered through the sliding glass door, and spotted me on the sofa. They weren't the same cops from last night, so at least I was spared that embarrassment.

They banged on the glass loudly. "Open the door!"

This time I was able to get up, stagger over to the sliding door, and let them in.

"Did you call 9-1-1?"

I nodded yes, although Mitch had called. I told them I had bipolar disorder, but I wasn't sure if they understood what that meant. They saw I was wearing only a pair of shorts.

"Don't you have any other clothes to put on? We're going to get an ambulance to take you to the hospital."

I motioned toward my upstairs bedroom. "I have a pair of sweatpants and a T-shirt in my dresser drawers."

One of the officers made his way upstairs and was able to find them. When he returned, he tossed them next to me on the couch.

"Put these on."

Thankfully, this all occurred during late morning hours on a weekday, so my neighbors were at work. Nobody witnessed the incident or heard my loud cries to Mitch to help me. They didn't see the police arriving at my doorstep or the ambulance whisking me away to the funny farm.

In the ambulance, I was given some type of relaxant, since I had continued to thrash. My next memory is waking up upon arrival at the psychiatric facility.

Inside the Psychiatric Ward (March 9, 2000)

According to the medical records that I obtained after my stay in the psych ward, I entered the emergency room at the hospital with the following admission evaluation: paranoid delusions, auditory hallucinations, suicidal ideation, and homicidal ideation toward an ex-coworker. I tried to convince my doctors that Jonathan was against me, leaving messages on my voicemail, and posting wacky pictures on the internet. He once told me he had photo shopped his own wife's head on a belly dancer as a joke. To this day, I'm not completely sure if he was simply pulling my leg, or if I was delusional.

Although I denied suicidal ideation, they told me I had written a suicide note. I had no recollection of this unless it pertained to my recent overdose of allergy pills that I had mistaken for sleeping pills. They determined my mood swings had been mixed from depression to euphoria. I had experienced poor appetite and inadequate sleeping. My speech was somewhat rapid with a flight of ideas. I had poor concentration and impaired memory.

My doctor asked, "Are you hearing voices in your head?"

"I'm hearing inspirations from God . . . and good and evil voices."

"Are you feeling paranoid?"

"I believe the CIA, FBI, and a government coworker are following me via a satellite, recording my conversations."

"Are you aware that you wrote a threatening warning to your friend, Jonathan?"

"He's not my friend. He was my coworker, and I want to kill him because he is posting pictures of me on the internet."

"Do you want to call your family and let them know you're here?"

"No, I don't want to call my family. Have my social worker do that."

The following day, I was agitated. "I was fine until two weeks ago—I know someone is after me, and I still would kill him." I said to my doctor in a cryptic tone.

Although I was referring to Jonathan, it could just as easily have been Arnie since I had threatened to take his life within the past forty-eight hours as well.

I became despondent over my situation. "I'm not suicidal. I'm just depressed that I have to be here . . . I know he is causing this problem."

During my stay, I underwent severe psychotic symptoms, including auditory hallucinations—hearing voices that nobody else could hear because they didn't exist. The grandiose delusions that I experienced were based on my beliefs that I was having conversations with God. I was then sharing these verbal inspirations with the three imaginary voices in my head.

Sonya, Cliff, and Priscilla, continued to occupy my thoughts. Each of my bipolar episodes had included "conversations" with one or more of them in my head. I had read this is common in bipolar disorder. As mentioned at the onset of my first episode, they were actual colleagues of mine with a former employer. Sonya was an attractive blonde. Cliff was a prematurely gray, philosophical man with a clever wit and playful sense of humor. Priscilla was an ex-manager of mine, whose opinion I respected and discourse I enjoyed. Our discussions were often deep and thought-provoking.

In my typical hallucination, I was a professor. The three of them sat in an otherwise empty amphitheater-style auditorium extending above me.

One night, our debate centered on whether Archie Manning was the greatest quarterback of all time. I argued that he was. They unanimously contended I was crazy. My hallucination would invariably end the same way, with me jumping high into the air, and whacking my head . . . against the ceiling of my cell. At least now I know why I had lumps on my head.

Mental illness, in my case at least, could be both comical and fascinating. At the end of one exchange, I believed that I visualized a colossal image of Pinocchio with a rubber hammer, hitting me over the head. The melody of Looney Tunes was playing loudly with the lyrics, "Thaaaat's all folks!" It left me wondering if there were others who have traveled back from the outer reaches of mental illness and delusions to share such bizarre accounts.

Another talk revolved around Noah's Ark. Was it folklore or reality? As all creationists and believers are convinced, the Bible clearly states that Noah and his sons built the ark while he preached repentance to the masses over a one hundred and twenty-year period. He warned of the world being destroyed by flood.

I reminded my audience of three that, back in Noah's time, it never rained. The ground was saturated by a morning mist or dew, similar to what still exists today. Noah's preaching fell on deaf ears. The people ridiculed his warning that water was going to pour down from the clouds since they could not even fully comprehend the concept of rain.

Sonya interrupted my monologue. "What proof is there to support your claim?"

"The Bible says that it rained for forty days and forty nights after Noah, his family and two of every living creature, one male and one female, entered the ark. When the waters that engulfed the entire planet subsided, the topology of the earth was restructured permanently."

Cliff chimed in. "You still haven't provided proof."

"Well, okay, for instance, creationists believe that the magnificent Grand Canyon was formed in the aftermath of the floods, that the sudden shifting as the waters subsided caused the incredible rock erosion."

"That's crazy!" said Priscilla. "Science teaches that the Grand Canyon was formed over billions and billions of years through gradual erosion from the Colorado River at the base of the canyon."

"Well science is wrong. According to the Bible, the earth is only about six thousand years old, and I believe through faith that every word is one hundred percent true."

"Yeah, *blind* faith," mocked Sonya.

"Steve, you're nuts," said Cliff. "Have you ever even been to the Grand Canyon?"

"No, but I plan on visiting someday. It's on my bucket list."

"I suppose you're going to preach to us now about fire and brimstone hailing from the sky and destroying the wicked on judgment day, right?" asked Priscilla, sounding annoyed.

"Actually, I wasn't, but, like the floodwaters that cascaded from above during Noah's day, it's entirely possible. It would certainly be unexpected; that's for sure."

After failing to reach closure on this debate, we moved on to the next topic. Undoubtedly, the most philosophical discussions of all centered on God. This is an underlying theme in my episodes.

"During my bipolar journey, I am convinced God has been speaking to me, and that I have been inspired in the same way as the various authors of the Bible."

"You're not serious, are you?" inquired Sonya. "You think God has been talking to you?"

"Really, that's a bit arrogant, don't you think?" added Priscilla.

"Why not? I've been speaking with you guys throughout my episodes, and I can't see or touch you, right?"

"Let's hear what Mister Prophet has to say about his actual conversation with God," Cliff said sarcastically.

"I am a huge fan of Van Morrison, although this wasn't always the case," I replied with a smile. "Except for "Brown-eyed Girl," of course, I was turned on to him in my late-thirties by a British coworker. I came to discover Van Morrison's music masterful. My favorite song is "Wavelength." As a songwriter myself for the better part of thirty-five years, it's one of the tunes I wish I had written. Well, God revealed "Wavelength" to me as a means to help me tackle one of the greatest riddles in life: How is He able to reside in everyone's heart, and soul, and mind at the same time, and listen to our thoughts and prayers, taking into account the more than 7.6 billion people on the planet Earth at present."

I paused to create suspense as they awaited my response.

"The obvious creationist answer is simple . . . because he is God. However, for those seeking a worldly explanation to solve this conundrum, I pondered the following hallucinatory revelation. Consider this basic analogy: We are all on different *spiritual* wavelengths with God. Like a transistor radio (as referenced in "Brown-eyed Girl"), we each have varying frequencies on the dial. My radio station might be W-E-S-T 888 FM. This unique frequency over the airwaves would be my direct signal to communicating with God. This format would continue throughout the entire world population since there would be an infinite number of spiritual frequency combinations available. "Is this making any sense, guys?""

"A little," they mumbled in unison.

"Okay, here is another example to advance my bipolar-induced theory. I worked at a major software corporation for a brief period during my career. I couldn't differentiate an end user software seat from a toilet seat. However, I did discover a few things while I was sitting there alone in my cubicle trying to look busy, contemplating the universe. My revelation about wavelengths was unveiled to me during a bipolar episode, which should help explain my mindset at the time. This is my disclaimer in case you think this sounds crazy."

"Please get to the point," said Priscilla.

"Host computer mainframes are like God. The remote computers they communicate with through the network cloud all have unique *addresses*. These individual identifiers allow them to have conversations with the host simultaneously. Unlike God, however, there are limitations as to how many physical devices can be connected to the internet. As it continues to rapidly evolve, this will become less of an issue. Personal computers, naturally, represent us. However, the internet will always be finite, whereas God, of course, is infinite. It actually does make some sense if you think about it."

As this hallucination ended, the room was quiet and I was drowsy, perhaps from the lumps on my head caused by Pinocchio's mallet and jumping. I waved my three comrades goodbye without a sound and drifted into a deep sleep. When I awoke from my dream, I discovered myself in the den of some old house. There was an oversized grand piano in the corner of the room. Van Morrison was wearing a top hat and tap dancing up and down the ivory keyboard playing the tune of "Wavelength" in the dark. It was like a scene out of *Alice in Wonderland*. The Bible was the only open book on the shelf. There were footsteps down the hall of someone coming to get me.

***

March 13, 2000

According to hospital records, when I was back in conversation with my doctor, my speech was rapid and stressful. "I have spent over a million dollars recording twenty-four Christian songs," I said in an obvious exaggeration.

At that point I had paid around twenty thousand dollars recording a compact disc of nineteen Christian songs because I felt certain that God was making spiritual revelations to me. In my mind, I was a sort of modern-day prophet.

Later, I spoke with my therapist concerning my fear of being crazy. "You can learn how to manage your illness," she said.

"I know. I still don't understand why I went off my medications. It was to please my girlfriend. She discovered my meds and questioned my need to take them."

"Why did you let her talk you into it?"

"She is a pharmacist so I thought she knew what was best for me. I was embarrassed and tried to hide them from her, then stopped taking them altogether."

"Now, have you learned from your mistake?" she asked.

"Yes, I realize the importance of taking my meds to help me function."

During a group session, I apologized for venting my desire earlier to hurt my coworker. "I wanted to get back at him financially for what he did to me. I don't know why I said those things about wanting to kill him. I have trouble even killing a mosquito."

It would be about ten days before I was well enough to finish in-house treatment and be on my way home. Time passed quickly, and soon I was planning for discharge. I was ready. "I feel like a million dollars!" I shouted to no one in particular while in group therapy as several heads turned my way in response to the commotion.

However, my jubilation was soon tempered with the realization that I had no job to return to. And, despite wanting to go home, the truth was that I had exhausted my health benefits and I had to leave before I probably should have.

During the final week of March, I headed home. The first thing I did was make an appointment with Lois, an attorney and a friend of my sister Linda. Lois was an evangelical Christian, so I figured I was in good hands. I asked her to send Glenn a letter to request a retraction of my resignation.

Her claim was that my appeal for termination was a misguided way of dealing with the stress of my illness. She elaborated that I enjoyed my job and had received consistent satisfactory performance reports from management. She included the advisement from my doctor to not resume work until April 3, 2000, at which time I expected to be fully recuperated.

Unfortunately, my remaining hopes were short-lived. My attorney received a letter from the vice-president of human resources dated March 28, 2000, containing the following reply:

---

*I am responding to your letter dated March 24, 2000, by which Mr. West
seeks to retract his written letter of resignation. Based upon all the facts in
connection with Mr. West's resignation, it is clear that Mr. West voluntarily
resigned his employment. We will not accept Mr. West's attempted retraction
of his resignation. In fact, Mr. West's threat of violence against our
employees is grounds for termination, whether or not he resigned.
We wish Mr. West success in his future endeavors.*

I was figuratively escorted to the door. The culprit was my bipolar
disorder, which had served to get me rudely, yet fairly in this case,
dismissed from a high-paying job.

(Note: On October 24, 2001, my lawyer received a copy of the
Order of Dismissal signed by the judge, which brought my
unsuccessful claim to a close.)

CLINICAL OVERVIEW (CHAPTER EIGHT)

*I*s *there a correlation between musical and artistic creativity and bipolar disorder?*

 In a large 2015 study, scientists in Iceland reported that genetic factors in bipolar disorder (BD) and schizophrenia are found more often in people in creative professions. Painters, musicians, writers and dancers were, on average, twenty-five percent more likely to carry the gene variants than less creative professions, such as farmers, manual laborers and salespeople.

The scientists drew on genetic and medical information from eighty-six thousand Icelanders. They found genetic variants that doubled the average risk of schizophrenia and raised the likelihood of bipolar disorder by more than one-third. When they looked at how common these variants were in members of national arts societies, they found a seventeen percent increase compared with the less creative members[26].

The researchers went on to check their findings in large medical databases in the Netherlands and Sweden. Among these thirty-five thousand people, those deemed to be creative (by profession or through answers to a questionnaire), were nearly twenty-five percent more likely to carry the mental disorder genes.

These are the primary studies that investigate rates of mood disorders in creative individuals using personal interviews of the subjects. They also involve a diagnosis that reflects modern concepts of depression and bipolar disorder. While they vary slightly in the lifetime prevalence rates reported, all results run in the same direction. Therefore, it seems likely that creative individuals do have higher rates of mood disorder in general, and bipolar disorder in particular. However, it is important to note that a limitation of these studies is that they have focused *primarily* on writers, to date.

There appears to be an association between creativity and mood disorder. Rates of mood disorder are extremely high in the writers; eighty percent had some type of mood disorder, and thirty percent of this subset group had either bipolar I or bipolar II disorder. These rates are significantly different from the control subjects[27].

Controlled quantitative studies and retrospective qualitative studies based on biographical research show that bipolar disorder occurs commonly in creative individuals. It is far less prevalent in the general population as a whole[28].

Katherine P. Rankin, Ph.D. and colleagues at the University of California-San Francisco stated, "It is well-established that people with affective disorders tend to be overrepresented in the creative artist population (especially those with bipolar disorder). Bipolar disorder may carry certain advantages for creativity, especially in those who have milder symptoms[29]."

CHAPTER NINE SECOND EPISODE – PART 5 APRIL 2000

I needed work. I had now been victimized for a second time by a major bipolar episode. I was still dealing with the consequences of foolishly coming off my medications. I touched upon this subject earlier, but it bears repeating. The actual hospitalizations of my episodes were similar to the epicenter of an earthquake. I discovered that the subsequent tremors or aftershocks could persist for months or even years depending on the level of treatment or lack thereof with proper medications I had received.

During this second episode, I discontinued my pills in a late July 1999 timeframe. Predictably, a short while later in August, my bipolar condition escalated significantly during my trip to Israel. Despite this manifestation, there were many mood cycles over the next eight months involving mania, despondency, heightened anger issues, and paranoia that surfaced and disappeared. Eventually, under an unbearable burden of stressful situations, I "crashed" and wound up hospitalized.

Now my friend Jerry had left the reseller where we'd worked together to start his own business. He was fulfilling his dream of becoming an entrepreneur. It was the year 2000, and dotcom companies were cropping up worldwide. Jerry's idea was to create a company catering to small businesses interested in setting up their own website. His startup would design and manage the websites in return for a nominal monthly charge. His plan made sense to me. It was a cutting edge idea in that his service would be one of the first of its kind in the industry. With this opportunity came big risk. Jerry didn't have a lot of capital dollars to play with so it was potentially hit or miss.

I had helped him on many occasions when I was his sales manager and had admittedly given him most of the better sales leads. This might be why he agreed to bring me on board his new venture. I was feeling very negative at the time, with no self-confidence whatsoever. Understandably, after suffering two major episodes, my nerves were shattered. Although I didn't know it yet, I would discover each passing episode was worse than the one before it.

Initially the business floundered. My first two paychecks bounced. He had given me the title of customer service manager, even though we didn't yet have any customers to manage. To drum up client activity, Jerry had set up a call center in Houston, Texas, where he located cheap labor. We flew there at least twice on business.

When we arrived at the center, the handful of employees I met appeared to be clueless. They seemed to need guidance and supervision on every detail involving customer service. This ranged from professionally interacting with a client on the telephone to resolving support issues. Jerry later confessed he was paying them over twenty thousand dollars more than me a year. I reconsidered. Maybe they weren't as clueless as I thought.

They were complaining about needing marketing training, and Jerry assured them I was their guy. They were beginning to get restless during our first meeting at the call center. They wanted answers. I had none to offer.

When we flew there for the second meeting shortly thereafter, he must have finally begun to sense something was still wrong with my mental state. He instructed me prior to our group gathering. "Just do what I do." Jerry and I were close friends, but he had to put his company first.

In fairness to him, I had never mentioned my recent hospitalization for obvious reasons. I didn't want to call his attention to my bipolar condition. In addition, I had been released prematurely from the hospital since my health insurance had expired with my recent job termination. Finally, a retrospective check of my medical records revealed that I was only functioning at a level 40 on a scale of 1 to 100 upon my release.

Jerry understandably told me to be quiet while he did the talking and training. He wore a pair of black shorts as we made the long drive from the airport to the call center. We were slated to meet with two or three supervisors and their telemarketers that afternoon.

I motioned to his shorts. "You're going to change, right?"

"I'm the president of the company, Westy."

"Exactly, which is why you should be wearing pants." I was able to convince him, and we found a strip mall along the way to make the switch.

The meeting was a disaster. I couldn't answer any questions. I did have a strong marketing background and would normally have performed without a hitch. But now my brain was shut down. I couldn't wait to get home. My depression was brought about by a combination of appearing incompetent as a result of my mental illness and knowing what I faced upon my arrival. Sure enough, I was let go not long after that. But a few interesting incidents happened before my dismissal.

One day, Jerry was particularly excited. He was always a very positive, upbeat kind of guy. He exclaimed, "Westy, I just heard about a can't-miss opportunity to make a fortune, and I want to let you in on it."

Naturally, I was all ears.

"A company is supposed to be going public that makes a state-of-the-art tire."

"Tire? Did you just say *tire*?" I asked incredulously as I popped up in my chair.

"It has a special tread to it, which allows it to grip the road so your car won't hydroplane in wet weather." He continued. "What do you think?"

"I think you're crazy." Here I was calling someone else crazy.

"The investment is ten thousand dollars, but we'll have to make the decision today."

I did have more than a hundred thousand dollars in savings and investments at the time, accumulated during my lucrative sales days. I wasn't typically a high-risk guy and I normally would have told him to get lost, but my mind was weak.

"What are you going to do, Jerry?"

"I think I'm going to go ahead with it."

I did, too. I invested ten thousand dollars, and I never saw a dime. What truly happened, I'll never know. I can barely even recall the incident. Only Jerry knows the details.

I still suspect to this day that something fishy occurred. I never did learn the name of this company with the supposed magical tires. I also found it a bit peculiar that he had ten thousand dollars to risk when he had already bounced my first two paychecks, and the new company was floundering. I must have been out of my mind to trust him.

Another strange incident happened when I told him I was a born-again Christian. He enthusiastically pulled open his top desk drawer.

"Get out. So am I!" He screamed in delight as he removed a notebook. "Every morning, I say a prayer and jot it down here in my book. It's my personal diary."

I admired Jerry for his words, but not for his actions. He wasn't even Christian, let alone evangelical.

Jerry fired me shortly thereafter. In case you're keeping score, my bipolar job terminations had now reached three, as I had been victimized once again. We stood just outside his front door in view of his wife when he delivered the bad news. I can't say I was surprised from a business standpoint. It was what later took place that grieves me to this day.

He eliminated me entirely from his personal life. Our friendship was over. I had lost another close friend because of my mental illness, just like I had lost Becky and Jonathan. Sadly, there would be more to follow. I called Jerry on multiple occasions, practically begging him to meet me for lunch at our favorite Chinese restaurant. He would agree at first, and then cancel only minutes before our arranged meeting time. Pathetically, it wouldn't even be from him, but rather his secretary.

"Hello, Steve," she would say. "I'm calling you from Jerry's office . . . he said to tell you he's sorry, but he can't make it today. Something came up. You'll have to do it some other time."

Then there were the times I called his office and his receptionist answered the phone.

"May I please speak with Jerry?" I inquired.

"May I ask who is calling?"

"Steve West."

"May I ask what this is in reference to?"

"Yes, I'm an old friend of his."

"Okay, Mr. West, please hold."

She returned to the line. "I'm sorry, Mr. West. Jerry's in a meeting. Can he call you back?"

"Yes, he has my number," I sighed.

I never heard back from him. I tried again on several other occasions, but it was always the same result. He didn't have time for me or he was in a meeting.

He obliges me by email when I ask for a work reference or recommendation. I'll give him that much. When I politely thank him, he always responds, "You don't have to thank me. I'm always happy to help you out."

Except he just doesn't want to talk to me. I almost sense he's afraid I would ask for my old job back. It's a situation that saddens me to this very day.

World Travel Episode(s) Late Summer 2000

After my short-lived career with Jerry's dotcom company, I needed a break from the action of trying to secure long-term employment, both physically and mentally. I had enjoyed the good fortune of visiting fifty-five countries on six continents throughout my lifetime. I had set foot on each of the continents at least three times. The one I have yet to traverse is Antarctica. I have experienced bipolar episodes in some of these places from mild to severe. The last of my overseas excursions was in the year two thousand to Buenos Aires, Argentina, and Costa Rica.

My photograph album triggers haunting memories of being over-medicated in the aftermath of episode two. I vividly recall riding a horse and almost falling from my mount. There is another picture of me attempting to swing on a vine. And another of me sitting on a wall and staring into space, a feat that I had mastered.

I continued onward to Costa Rica, to its magnificent and world-renowned rain forest. I scaled it by cable car with a couple who were on their honeymoon. They snapped photographs of the fantastic, dew-drenched scenery, greenery, and the like. As for me? I slept the whole way.

Although I enjoy travel, I couldn't simply leave my mental illness behind. For example, I embarked on several Windjammer voyages and on one of the trips, I never left my cabin. At first, I had hoped it was seasickness, but I had sailed enough to know this unfortunately was not the case. I had foolishly set sail while undergoing a bipolar episode.

I was too crazed to see anyone. I had a roommate who understandably didn't like me because of how I acted. Neither did anyone else on the small wooden ship. It was really tight quarters for anyone, but especially someone undergoing an acute attack of paranoia and depression. There were only about seventy-five passengers on board the tiny ship.

One of them was an attractive woman whom I initially was trying to impress during a brief visit on deck from my subterranean cabin. Unfortunately, she saw right though my guise. She leaned on one of the rails of the small ship when I sauntered over with a bottle of beer. The captain was scaling to the top of the mast pole to untangle the sails that had gotten snared in the violent wind gusts. I told her I was going to climb up there with him to lend a hand.

"No, you won't," she mocked.

"Why not?" I inquired.

"Because you're not that type of personality, and you seem very strange."

This remark made me even more uncomfortable, so I excused myself abruptly and retreated to the safety of my cabin.

Midway to the beautiful British Virgin Island of Tortola in the Caribbean Sea east of Puerto Rico, I had to ask the captain to have me taken ashore by medical personnel to visit a hospital. There were still several days left on our voyage and I was uncertain that I would make it. It was the most primitive hospital I have ever encountered in my life, but what was to be expected on a small island? Basically, they gave me some aspirin, took my temperature and blood pressure, and I was on my way.

Not too surprisingly, they failed to test me for bipolar disorder.

The most embarrassing moment of the whole ordeal was being escorted to shore in a small boat. I had hoped to escape while the other passengers were still away on the beach in order to avoid additional humiliation. Unfortunately, they were returning from their all-day snorkeling and scuba diving excursion. I was the only one who hadn't joined this typically fun-filled experience. When the two boats passed, I heard laughter, which I assumed was at my expense.

I put myself up in a hotel for the night on the island, which wound up being in the middle of nowhere. I didn't recover any of the money for my three remaining days of the trip. Shortly after, Windjammer went out of business. My three voyages over the years were not enough to sustain them.

By the turn of the century, my international travel days came to a sudden halt, largely because of my bipolar disorder. My financial situation was worsening as well since I had now lost several high-paying jobs. Lastly, my burning desire to travel abroad was flickering as I had seen all the distant places I had envisioned in my life. It was time for me to turn my attention closer to home and to get my health back in order.

Winter 2000 Street Preaching

After losing my job, I suddenly had a lot of free time to myself. My brother, Tim, and his friends had decided to initiate a part-time street ministry on weekends. They set up speakers in the back of their van in the heart of New York City, and took turns preaching for hours to the masses about the virtues of seeking Christianity. They faced intense confrontation from passers-by of various conflicting religions. On multiple occasions, my outspoken brother would admonish these opponents with harsh verbal exchanges that nearly resulted in physical altercations. The police, who had provided us with our permit, were always close at hand to maintain the peace.

One of Tim's cohorts pleaded with the small crowd that had gathered on the street corner, "Listen to me, people, you're going to hell if you don't get saved."

Tim and his friends constantly tried to coax me into grabbing the microphone and joining them in their spiritual warfare against the wicked world, but, I always balked. I was too frightened by the potential backlash and embarrassment I might face if a friend or acquaintance caught me preaching the word of God. I was still a mess when involved in stressful situations because of my bipolar disorder.

One stranger approached me and asked incredulously, "Are you with these guys?" I felt certain this was in reference to my quiet demeanor and low-key approach to what was taking place on the nearby corner. My brother was screaming into the microphone for all the sinners to repent.

After debating whether I should deny that I was with the group as the apostle Peter did in the Bible when asked if he were with Jesus, I decided to be honest. "Yes," I said.

He shook his head in amazement and continued down the block.

I decided to limit my participation in our street preaching ministry to the handing out of Christian tracts to anyone who would accept them. Most of the pamphlets wound up in trash cans or littering the sidewalks of midtown Manhattan. I also carried a large box filled with my spiritual compact discs containing the nineteen songs that I had recently recorded at the studio. Although it was free, the CD entitled *"Go to Heaven,"* was also regularly rejected. It saddened me that we were unable to convince them to accept a complimentary gift simply because it pertained to Jesus.

After an arduous day of street preaching, we would typically visit one of the group's houses for dinner. Tim and his friends were convinced my bipolar condition was the work of demons that needed to be cast out. He and his friends were determined to cure me of my demonic mental illness permanently. They took turns laying hands on me, just like in the Bible. I felt the whole situation was wacky, but in my weakened state of mind I agreed to give it a try. It failed miserably. I spit up a few times into a garbage can in an effort to rid myself of the demons through vomiting. Then I hurried home to take my bipolar meds before I lost my sanity.

Our gang eventually dispersed. Tim married one of the women in the group and relocated to Florida. Other members paired up as well, and went their separate ways. Before he left, there was a front page article in the state's largest newspaper about Tim and his local street preaching.

Unable to Find Work

During the latter part of 2000, I was unable to secure employment. I flitted between job opportunities at a whirlwind pace in an effort to discover something promising. Having lost Jonathan as a friend, I no longer had anyone to endorse me to high-level hiring managers. My friend Jerry, at least, was willing to provide references and letters of recommendation, but it was difficult to communicate with him via telephone since he didn't make himself available. For eighteen years now, all our correspondence has been by email, which is disheartening.

Still reeling from the aftereffects from episode two, I met with rejection at every doorstep. An employment agency arranged an interview for me with a well-known software company. I was ushered into the conference room where I was to be briefed by one of the president's staff prior to my upper level meeting with him. I had come highly recommended because of my successful career at the major software corporation where I had attained sales support recognition. We appeared to be a good match. Unfortunately, I was not at my best—to say the least.

"Can I get you some coffee or bottled water?" he inquired.

Trying my best to stay focused, I stared into space.

"Are you familiar with our organization and product line?"

Avoiding eye contact, I tried in vain to collect my scattered thoughts.

"Do you have any questions for me before you meet the president?"

Shifting uneasily in my seat, I dried my moist palms on my suit pants.

He excused himself and stormed out of the room, slamming the door in the process. When he returned, he claimed the president was in a meeting, and turned his back to me, clearly agitated. He escorted me to the front exit without even a handshake. I had wasted his time and, more importantly, the president's time who had scheduled the appointment to see me.

Then there was another instance when I was able to obtain an interview at a small data communications firm in New York City. I had no interest in struggling with the daily commute, but I was desperate for work. The group meeting was going well, as I was being questioned by three executives. Then they dropped the bomb.

"We're a tight-knit business here. Our families socialize after work; we get together for barbeques and other events. We're a very family-oriented company. Are you married?"

A bell immediately rang in my head. I had been cautioned a hundred times that this was an illegal question to be asked of a prospective employee at an interview. What should I do? I sat there agonizing as the three pairs of eyes stared at me, anxiously awaiting my response.

"No, I'm not married. I'm divorced."

After a short pause, one of them replied, "Oh, so you're just a single bachelor, out there playing the field."

I knew my position was hopeless. They were wrong for behaving like they did. The question *was* illegal, as was their unprofessional and ignorant retort to my candid admission. But, what could I do? The reality of the situation was that small, privately run organizations have no human resources department in which to file a complaint. And, in my current state-of-mind, I had no desire to file a lawsuit.

The rejection kept mounting. My confidence had tumbled into a bottomless pit of despair. A customer service company turned me away because I didn't have a good telephone voice. I was shown the door at another small telecom firm even though I knew the director from a previous employer. He said the reason was because my training supervisor didn't feel I was qualified for the position. I was offered a role selling frozen meat and other food delicacies door-to-door on a straight commission basis. Unfortunately, I lasted only one day before being chased from an owner's property during a sales visit. Apparently, my timing was terrible; I had interrupted an important long-distance telephone conversation. He was furious when he discovered the purpose of my call, and I scurried down the block with my wares.

I decided to call Priscilla. Yes, the same one whose imaginary, episodic voice would sometimes penetrate my brain along with Sonya and Cliff. Only now, she was quite real. Priscilla was a mid-level manager at the large telecommunications company where I was once employed. Although I had known her for years, I could barely control my voice from cracking during my long-winded message seeking her assistance.

She returned my call promptly and was polite, even though she could sense my desperation.

"Is everything okay, Steve? You sound like you're nervous."

"Actually, I'm out of work, and was wondering if there were any openings for selling telephone systems." I was glad she couldn't see my hand trembling on the handset.

"I'm sorry, but the big emphasis today is on data communications and the internet. When you were here awhile back, they were still new to our product line. I'm not sure you'd be a good fit now."

"Oh, that's okay," I answered, feeling deflated. "I understand. Can I still use you as a job reference, at least?"

"Of course. Not a problem."

I'd been having a hard time obtaining three references, even from former colleagues and friends. I assumed they were starting to question my competency because of my inability to keep a job.

Even my aunt and uncle who were visiting from Florida at the time admonished me.

"You're pale as a ghost. What are you on dope?" she asked.

"I wouldn't hire you if I were a company. You look like a zombie!" he added.

The fact was, I was over-medicated.

Finally, after all the rejection, I wound up accepting a temporary position for a telemarketing group. We collected money from parishioners of a local church to pay for the enhancement of the facility. Somehow, I lasted there part-time for three months. I had now officially worked *every* menial job in my life, including newspaper delivery, washing dishes, selling pots and pans, stocking supermarket shelves, loading trucks, and selling buttons.

CLINICAL OVERVIEW (CHAPTER NINE)

W*here can you locate information to help educate your friends and the public about bipolar disorder?*
Most folks have heard about bipolar disorder (BD) and may know a loved one, friend or coworker who suffers from the disease. Like most other mental illnesses, there is a stigma attached to BD because those who suffer from it have no way to defend themselves. The stigma derives from society's belief that those with mental illness are either psychopaths or intellectually disabled. People often generalize mood swings as BD. It is critical to educate the public about this serious condition, which attracts far too much negative press in our society.

Gabe Howard is an award-winning writer, activist, and speaker who lives with bipolar and anxiety disorders. According to Howard, below is the best information to share with those who might know someone with this dreaded mental disease.

"Bipolar disorder is a spectrum of moods that goes from the lowest of lows (suicidal_depression) all the way up to the highest of highs ("god-like" mania), and everything in between. The person suffering from bipolar is unable to control where their moods fall on this spectrum, or how long that mood will last before transitioning[30]."

BD is a severe and persistent mental illness with a fifteen percent death rate. Typical symptoms include racing thoughts (which lead to hurried and nonsensical speech); rapid mood swings, ranging from depression all the way to mania; staying awake for days at a time without tiring; and grandiose thinking, such as believing you have more fame, money, or authority than you really do.

"BD is an illness that affects the mind. Specifically, it alters a person's ability to govern their thoughts, behaviors, and the way they see the world around them. Someone suffering from bipolar will travel back and forth on a very long mood spectrum that they cannot control. This includes those that the average person will never experience, such as suicidal thoughts[31] or living in a consequence-free environment where a person feels invincible."

The Depression and Bipolar Support Alliance (DBSA)[32] is the leading peer-directed national organization focusing on the two most prevalent mental health conditions, depression and bipolar disorder, which together affect more than twenty-one million Americans. These two illnesses account for ninety percent of the nation's suicides every year, and cost twenty-three billion dollars in lost workdays and other workplace losses.

DBSA has nearly six hundred and fifty support groups and more than two hundred and fifty chapters. They reach millions of people each year with in-person and online education peer support. What's different about DBSA?

- They are peer-led. More than half of their staff and board members live with a mood disorder and all support groups are facilitated by peers.
- Focus is solely on bipolar disorder and depression.
- Nationally recognized for their mental health advocacy work.
- Innovative. They provide leading-edge, interactive online resources.

- Wellness-centered. DBSA informs, empowers, supports, and inspires individuals to achieve the lives they want to lead.

In short, DBSA provides hope, help, support, and education to improve the lives of people who have mood disorders.

There are many other services and treatment options that may provide assistance if you or someone you know is struggling with a mental illness. One such support group is the National Alliance on Mental Illness (NAMI)[33]. There are more than nine hundred and fifty NAMI Affiliates in communities across the country that can educate you about your symptoms and diagnosis.

THIRD EPISODE

CHAPTER TEN THIRD EPISODE – PART 1 MY TRIP TO NEW ORLEANS

In February 2001, I landed a job, my sixth in six years. My resume was a mess, appearing as though I was hopping from company to company with reckless abandon. I still had some jitters, and sporadic traces of my second bipolar episode seemed to be around every corner. I had made it through a bizarre interviewing process, with the hiring manager surveying my checkered credentials, asking me one or two questions to which I mumbled barely audible, incoherent responses. Still, he offered me the job.

The new employer was a pipe manufacturing firm. I had been hired at an embarrassingly low initial salary compared to my previous jobs. I began in the sales department and failed miserably for four or five months, until I was mercifully transferred to the product support group, where I had the daily responsibility of handling customer service technical issues. Although I had very little product knowledge, I managed to prevail. The first year passed without any major incidents.

In the summertime of 2002, an interesting event happened. Upper management asked me to attend an industry trade show convention in New Orleans. This exhibition provided vendors with the opportunity to display their product line to potential wholesale dealers and distributors. I would work the booth with my three colleagues, Chad, Donnie, and Jimmy.

As soon as I heard the venue was in New Orleans, an ulterior motive presented itself. I had already encountered my boyhood idol, Archie Manning, on multiple occasions during my hallucinatory bipolar episodes. This might be my golden chance to meet and chat with him in the flesh.

My supervisor had recently left our company and his office was temporarily empty. I gathered the courage to slip into it unnoticed a week before the trade show to carry out my scheme. I dialed the operator and asked for the telephone exchange for New Orleans.

"What party are ya'll trying to reach?" she drawled.

I hesitantly replied, "Archie Manning."

There was a short pause: "The football player?"

"Yes, please."

"Okay, please hold for the number."

I was shocked. He had a listed number! (I later discovered he ran a consulting business and booked speaking engagements.) My palms were like sponges as I scribbled the number on a piece of paper. I frantically pondered what message I would leave on his answering machine. I dialed the number, and it picked up on the first ring.

"Hello, Archie Manning."

My heart was racing, and my mind was rambling, as I did my best impersonation of Ralph Kramden from the Honeymooners.

"H-h-h-h-h-hello, Archie. My name is Steve West." My voice continued to stutter over my words. "I'm from New Jersey. You don't know me, but I'm a big fan of yours. I'm going to be in New Orleans next week, and I thought maybe I could come by and get your autograph . . . I mean my autograph . . . I mean your autograph, please?"

"Sure, when ya'll planning on coming down, bud?"

I gave him the three dates, and he told me he would be out of town for the first two days at speaking engagements. However, he expected to be back by the afternoon of the final day. We agreed I would try to connect with him then.

***

The following week, the four of us arrived in the Crescent City. We doubled up on rooms. I shared one with Jimmy. Chad and Donnie occupied another. My loud snoring kept Jimmy awake all night. He wound up having to skip his shift manning the booth the first day because he slept in. The meds I had been taking since my second bipolar episode had resulted in a significant weight gain of at least twenty-five pounds, which didn't help my diagnosed sleep apnea.

One night, we cruised the renowned Bourbon Street on foot. After devouring several Po-boy submarine sandwiches and some filet gumbo, we hit the town. Our first order of business was to pick up some bead necklaces for future use. Of all the many clubs and joints available, my friends chose a dive bar. Donnie and Jimmy foolishly started downing shots and dancing with the girlfriends of the local rowdies.

I was unable to drink because of my bipolar meds, and I immediately sensed trouble in the situation with my friends anyway. I followed Chad outside to the bar's balcony, overlooking Bourbon Street. We each had a generous supply of bead necklaces in hand. True to custom, as the beautiful women would strut by below, they would raucously holler, "Throw us some beads!" In return, they would lift their shirts and flash us. I never had engaged in such bizarre entertainment in my somewhat sheltered life. I had discovered a new game. Many ladies had over a dozen "trophies" around their necks. All good things must come to an end, and I soon exhausted my supply of beads.

Meanwhile, Donnie and Jimmy were still out on the dance floor twirling their partners. As Chad and I reentered the bar, Donnie decided to buy the two flirtatious girls drinks. While he was doing so, one girl's boyfriend tapped him on the shoulder. When Donnie turned around, the guy sucker punched him, giving him a bloody lip.

Jimmy began to holler, "That's fucked up! That's fucked up!"

Somebody called the police, who arrived on the scene within minutes. Donnie decided not to press charges.

***

Later in the week, the four of us drove to a customer site to visit one of our major distributors in the area, Barry. He served us a seafood lunch along the waterfront. Instead of simply peeling my shrimp, I grabbed a fork and knife and began to cut them in half.

One of my coworkers teased me, "Didn't anyone ever teach you how to eat shrimp?"

They all laughed at my expense. The sad truth was that my mind had started to wander unexpectedly, and I had difficulty concentrating. Focus troubles due to my bipolar disorder had once again came on without warning.

That evening, Barry treated us to an excursion around the bay in a small fishing boat. Lost in thought, I didn't utter a word throughout our one-hour sail. Finally, I snapped out of my trance when one of my colleagues mentioned to Barry that I hoped to meet up with Archie Manning to get his autograph.

"You're wasting your time," said Barry. "Manning's not gonna have time to fuck with you."

Everybody chuckled, but I knew that I would have the last laugh.

POLAR EXTREMES

***

On the last day of the trade show, my coworkers and I dismantled our display booth. There was only about a two-hour window before I had to head to the airport. Suddenly filled with manic-induced energy, I sprinted back to our hotel with my briefcase in hand. When I had checked out that morning, I had left my suitcase with the concierge for safekeeping. As luck would have it, our hotel was situated directly across the street from the convention center. Even more amazing, Manning's business office was located in the atrium tower, which was part of the hotel as well. I flopped down on a couch in the lobby and made an anxious call.

He told me to come on up, where I was immediately confronted by his snarling secretary. Since I was unannounced, she was guarding her client from being accosted by aggressive fans. But Archie assured her it was okay and rose politely to greet me. Naturally, I had brought my cumbersome camera along with me in hopes of getting a snapshot of us together.

"Sue, can you do me a favor and take our picture?" He asked his secretary.

She stood slowly from behind her desk in the room outside Manning's office. By now, she was shooting daggers at me, but she obliged. Just for good measure, I asked her to snap a second photograph in case the first one didn't take.

I gathered that was my hint to leave; however, I sat down on the chair opposite him at his desk instead. My manic spree continued. He was signing colored photos of himself from his playing days as giveaways to his fans. He glanced at me quizzically when I asked him to autograph one for me. I requested his signature on a copy of his autobiography, of course, which I just happened to have with me.

Now he was shifting uneasily in his seat. Perhaps he was concerned I was a serial stalker. I was talking very rapidly, overstaying my welcome and attempting to engage him in small talk. "So, do you think the Saints have a chance at making the playoffs this year?"

"I don't know. We'll have to wait and see, bud," he replied.

Finally, I checked my watch and realized I had to hurry to catch my flight. When I got home, I immediately had the 4" x 6" pictures developed and enlarged into 8" x 10" size. I placed them in a self-addressed stamped envelope and mailed them to him to request his autograph. He didn't disappoint me. The photographs arrived in the mail a few days later. The pictures serve as a constant reminder of the few moments I spent with my boyhood idol. The inscriptions read, "To Steve, All my best. Archie Manning."

***

The following year the president of the manufacturing company called me into his office for a big assignment, undoubtedly unaware that I was now navigating my way around Pluto. I could barely concentrate or stay focused on what he was saying, let alone respond coherently.

He explained we had a former manufacturing plant in Denison, Texas, which was the birthplace of one of our most revered presidents, Dwight D. Eisenhower. The locals were eager to convert it into a tourist attraction, because it was an eyesore from the main highway. My role was to solicit a bid from a local company to test the grounds for asbestos dust or contaminants associated with its twenty-five-year manufacturing history. I was further instructed to conduct a local town council meeting with the concerned parties.

The meeting was very successful, and everyone complimented me on a job well done. The result was a nominal price quote of fifteen thousand dollars to perform the necessary testing. Fifteen thousand dollars for a billion dollar company. Once again, despite my mental illness, I had prevailed. I headed home to New Jersey proud of my accomplishment.

But my ecstasy was short-lived. When I circulated the internal document for approval, it was given the thumbs-up by everyone except our president. I sent him an email insisting he was wrong.

I sent the president of the company an email insisting he was wrong! And he didn't fire me. I persisted, and we got into an email battle.

I showed one of my sisters the email thread, and she gasped in horror.

"Oh my God. You sent him that? He's going to fire you!"

But, he never did. I wound up having seven lives, one for each year I was with the company.

He always sent emails in upper case to convey anger. Our final exchange ended with the following terse message:

"EFFECTIVE IMMEDIATELY YOU ARE NO LONGER ASSIGNED TO THIS PROJECT!"

In retrospect, I still can't understand why he didn't terminate me. The only plausible explanation is that all the other senior managers in the company supported my viewpoint. I obviously would have adopted a different approach if not for my uncontrollable mental condition at the time. This example represented another display of my blatant disrespect for authority figures.

Not so amazingly, he never did speak to me again. There was one comical instance when we both happened to be leaving the office at the same time. He stepped into the open elevator. When I entered with him, he stepped out of the elevator and pushed the button to send me down without him.

Switching Medications

It was in February 2003 when my condition took another turn for the worse. During a visit with my psychiatrist, he told me about a new medication on the market, a preferred alternative to my current mood stabilizer, since it promoted weight loss. He encouraged me to give it a shot. What did I have to lose?

Well, it turned out I had a lot to lose, including my sanity. Since I was gradually weaned off my existing mood stabilizer, the decompensation process was slow. Soon, I started to feel very strange. My thoughts were distracted; my nerves were unraveling; paranoia was setting in. It was that same unmistakable feeling I had experienced during my first two episodes in 1996 and 1999. By late March, my previous drug that promoted weight gain was out of my system entirely. I didn't realize it at the time, but this new drug was apparently incompatible with my other meds and causing them to "clash." Trouble was waiting around the corner. I was starting to slip away.

Around this time period, I underwent two sleep studies to address my issues with sleep apnea and snoring. This malady was keeping me awake at night, and my restlessness was resulting in extreme tiredness during the day. A second study was required because I was unable to fall asleep during the first attempt. While preparing for the initial procedure, the nurse attached several sensor "patches" to the area surrounding my brain. I felt that she was acting sinister and would attempt to read my mind as part of the testing. I suspected that she would install a microchip in my head once I dozed off for future tracking purposes. Although the study was unsuccessful, I was fitted for a CPAP (Continuous Positive Airway Pressure) breathing device.

I participated in the second study shortly thereafter with much better results. During this procedure, I was more relaxed. I perceived the hospital staff to be friendly, which made me comfortable. I enjoyed a full night's sleep with the CPAP device. Without it, my apnea and snoring were off the charts with a rating of ten on a scale of one to ten.

Although the nurse was one of the "good" people during this pleasant, successful study, I still maintained the notion that I was being fitted for a microchip. This would allow for their future ability to read my mind.

***

Weekly Support Groups

It was around this time that I attended a weekly mental illness support group. These private meetings were a place for people like me, who felt the need to guard our bipolar diagnoses. Unfortunately, mental illness carries a stigma and everyone was wary of being exposed.

We agreed as a group that the ignorant comment "*He (or she) is bipolar,*" was just that. Ignorant. After all, you would never refer to someone who had a serious physical ailment such as cancer with the phrase:

"He (or she) is cancer." Would you?

The correct terminology, of course, is:

"He (or she) has cancer . . . and "He (or she) has bipolar disorder."

Possibly the clearest observation from those gatherings was the realization that there are a lot of people worse off than me. Sometimes there can be a tendency to feel like you're suffering alone. The meetings helped remind me that I wasn't.

I often arrived straight from work in a suit and tie, after a day in the corporate world. Most everyone else would be dressed in sneakers and jeans. I stuck out like a banker in a dive bar. We would proceed around the group and share our experiences with bipolar disorder and/or depression. There was always someone who served as the monitor to ensure the meeting remained on track. He (or she) was responsible for controlling disorderly conduct if a member became unruly.

One evening, a brawny, fidgety, male group member, who appeared to be "juiced up" on his meds leaped out of his chair. Apparently provoked about an innocent remark from the person next to him, he issued a challenge. "You wanna dance . . . I'll dance," he shouted, raising his fists.

Several other members jumped in, grappled with him, and ushered him to the door. This was a reminder that people were in varying stages of mental illness recovery. But instances like this were extremely rare.

Some of the stories were sad while others contained humor. The important thing is they were all tales of normal people from everyday walks of life. We shared the common malady of mental illness. One member related a story about driving all the way to Canada for no reason other than an internal voice prodded him to do so. He made it to the Canadian border only to be stopped for not having a passport . . . or even a driver's license.

We discovered at a later meeting that a woman in the group, perhaps intrigued by his story, had moved in with him.

At the end of these gatherings, we passed the hat and everyone who could afford it contributed a dollar toward payment for the use of the room. Then we all disappeared back into society until we met up again the following week.

My Major Manic Attack

At the onset of my third episode, I also suffered with severe mania. I embarked upon an ill-advised, costly spending spree for no apparent reason. I own well over one hundred fifty compact discs, one hundred of which were purchased during my unexpected manic attack. I visited every record store in all the malls in the surrounding area and purchased CDs at a frantic pace. In fact, my total estimated expenditure was twelve hundred dollars.

Perhaps the craziest thing in all this madness was the need I felt to have at least one CD for every band on the store shelves, whether I liked them or not. For example, I wound up buying the CDs of *Red Hot Chili Peppers, Nine Inch Nails* and *Eminem*. These were artists I didn't even listen to. I couldn't name a single song. Still, I felt the urgent need to have them in my collection.

The other extreme held true as well. Concerning masterful artists such as Van Morrison, whose music I had only recently discovered, I now had a burning desire to own *every* CD he had ever recorded. I was able to locate about twenty, even though there were many more. My credit card bill skyrocketed that month.

But, there's so much more to this story. I visited several liquor stores over the following month. In 1996, during my first attempt at suicide, I had concocted a mixture of alcohol in a blender. Later, I discarded the bottles to eliminate any future temptation. Now, I decided to replenish my stock. I purchased a bottle of virtually every liquor known to mankind, including rum, whiskey, bourbon, vodka, gin, tequila, vermouth, Sambuca, and a dozen others. The only alcoholic beverage I drank other than beer was rum, so the rest were just for show. This increased my tab another three hundred dollars.

Next, I discovered eBay, and I wandered around this online database looking for bargains. Since Archie Manning, the former quarterback of the New Orleans Saints, was my boyhood role model, I typed his name in the search engine. I found a startling number of items for bidding and sale, many of them of great interest to me. There was an official game jersey from his rookie season in 1971 that was being offered for five hundred dollars. Naturally, I decided to bid on it. This was even though I already owned three of his jerseys, two of them being authenticated by the National Football League. The bidding price continued to soar. Fortunately, I was eventually outbid by some other fanatic.

I set my sights on 8" x 10" color and black and white Manning photographs. I was surprised at the number available, around twenty. I bid on every one of them. Successfully. Most of them were from his professional days, others from Ole Miss where he played in college.

Let's not forget his football trading cards. I walked away with approximately fifteen of them. I even scored a miniature statue of him, which I have on display at home. Altogether, including a few photographs of Van Morrison and Michele Pfeiffer, my eBay expenditures amounted to about five hundred dollars. My credit card bill continued to soar over two thousand dollars, with only the touch of a computer keyboard!

But, wait, there's more. I have always been infatuated with statues. In addition to my shot glass collection, where I have purchased more than one hundred and eighty along the way, I have procured miniature statues as well.

I was now living in a townhouse, and I decided on a whim to seek some outdoor statues for my front lawn and back deck. The local retail store had a small collection of dwarves, and I purchased several for my front lawn. I forgot about the landscapers who mowed the lawns at our complex on a weekly basis.

My dwarves were in their way, so they simply tossed them to the side to get their job done. It became obvious to me that I was being a pest, but it took several instances of the groundskeepers abusing my dwarves before I finally caught on that I needed a new strategy.

As my manic episode continued over several weeks, my statue collection expanded rapidly. I now had three cats, one bear (designed to hold a flower pot), a dog, a squirrel, a chipmunk, a giant turtle that connected to a garden hose and spouted water out of his mouth, and a hen or a rooster . . . I forget which.

I also seriously pondered purchasing a giant cascading water fountain that displayed five or six otters, to place along the driveway I shared with my neighbor, Carol. (The fountain cost more than eight hundred dollars.) When I ran the idea by her, she immediately balked, claiming it would attract mosquitos. I briefly contemplated the idea of simply moving it inside my living room, but changed my mind. Carol was my voice of reason, and over the years we became close friends since she and her husband, Shaun, always watched over me.

My crème de la crème came when I saw a life-size pink statue of a pig at a novelty store. I knew that I must have it to add to my growing collection. It cost over one hundred dollars. It was so heavy and bulky the store manager had to assist me in getting it to my car. I somehow lugged it to my front yard where I strategically hid it behind one of the bushes. But it turned out it wasn't out of harm's way. I'm convinced the landscapers deliberately shoveled dirt on it even though it was not on the lawn or in their path.

Carol would approach me from time to time with a bewildered expression on her face, presumably befuddled by my sudden fondness of animals. "So, how are your little friends doing today?"

"Actually, I'm strongly considering starting a collection for my back deck as well."

At this time, Carol was unaware of my bipolar disorder. She would learn about it shortly thereafter in June 2003 at the onset of my third episode, and this craziness would begin to make sense to her.

True to my word, I began designing my deck with additional statues. Only this time they weren't animals. The new theme was people. I had found a store on the highway that sold high-quality white stone statues. There were replicas of women adorned in old-fashioned clothing. One was holding a lantern. Another was riding on the back of an animal. There was one of a boy and girl kissing on a swing. They had been designed in the style of the Victorian Age. In total, there were half a dozen large statues on my back deck. There was barely enough room for me to sit in a reclining chair.

I also felt the need to rescue some of my animals in the front yard from the groundskeepers to save them from their ongoing abuse, so I relocated them to the back deck. I had already installed three wind chimes to eliminate any free air space. It was now so cluttered, I felt as though my privacy was being invaded, and I was constantly being watched by the statues.

One evening Carol ambled over from next door to observe where I was busy arranging them in order like soldiers. "I tried to buy some statues at the place you recommended to me, but they were all sold out. I guess you must have bought out the whole lot." She seemed a bit miffed.

I felt genuinely embarrassed and sympathetic. "I'll tell you what. I feel really bad, so would it make it any better if I gave you one of mine? You can have your choice."

Her countenance changed. "All right, I'll take the bear you have out front. I'll use it to hold one of my flower pots."

"Okay, you got it. It's yours."

She walked away happy, as I counted my latest monetary losses during my manic spree: another one thousand dollars easily! This brought my debt to over three thousand dollars in a matter of weeks.

My next purchase was for one of my niece's birthday. I knew she liked cats. I wandered into a Hallmark store at the mall one night and saw a collection of mid-size statues of cats in various comical poses. There were fifteen on display, each valued at about forty dollars. I bought one for her as a present . . . and the other fourteen for myself. Add another six hundred dollars to my tab.

I finished my spending spree with buying statues of the Three Stooges, pewter statues, miniature statues of every animal in creation, and a much larger, expensive statue of a wolf. Not to mention the four stepping stones engraved with grasshoppers, mice and other colorful animals, which I used to adorn the tiny dirt path leading to my front door. Statues, statues, statues! Altogether, my bipolar mania had added four thousand dollars to my credit card bill within that short period of time.

I culminated my manic attack by staying up until three in the morning the following night hammering nails into my garage wall. Naturally, I woke up every neighbor on the block. I had been rummaging through old boxes when I found over a dozen baseball caps. I decided to hang them up in the middle of the night because I couldn't sleep. Although I was clearly sleep-deprived for days, I still was able to function at a high energy level. Unfortunately, my next-door neighbors, including Carol and Shaun, weren't. They called me one night and angrily ordered me to cut it out.

CLINICAL OVERVIEW (CHAPTER TEN)

*H**ow can a caregiver assist a patient who has experienced a change in lifestyle or job loss because of bipolar disorder?*

When a patient has bipolar disorder, the first and most important thing is to assist them with is getting the right diagnosis and treatment. An appointment should be made to accompany them to visit the doctor. Encourage the patient to stay under the care of a therapist.

To help a friend or relative:

- Offer emotional support, understanding, patience, and encouragement.
- Learn about bipolar disorder so you can understand what they are experiencing.
- Listen to feelings they express to identify situations that may trigger bipolar symptoms.
- Invite them out for positive distractions, such as walks, outings, and other activities.
- Remind them that, with time and treatment, they will get better.
- Never ignore comments about your friend or relative harming themselves. Always report such comments to their therapist or doctor[34].

The loss of a permanent, well-paying job is one of the worst things that can happen to someone with mental illness. First, it means direct loss of income, perhaps the main source of money in the family. Second, it may include loss of medical insurance, which may be badly needed in the weeks and months ahead. Third, it equates to an unsatisfactory performance rating in one's personnel file, which may limit their chances of finding further employment. Fourth, it is a serious blow to the self-esteem of a depressive, whereas a manic may not even consider the loss worth notice because of grandiose delusion.

Most people do not have sufficient savings to face a prolonged period without income, and available funds are usually quickly exhausted. Soon, the rent or mortgage becomes overdue, and eviction follows. These difficulties are all magnified and accelerated if the victim is the principal wage-earner for a family. In such cases, the role and value of the person as an effective spouse or parent erodes quickly, and a separation or divorce can ensue. To make matters worse, there is almost no effective public assistance available to a seriously mentally ill person and his/her family. To obtain social security disability status can take months or even a year, and the benefit, once it starts, is minimal. It is barely enough if the ill person is the "guest" of another family member, but totally inadequate for even basic survival of an individual. This downward spiral is the reason so many mentally ill victims wind up as street people in our big cities, unable to help themselves in any way that will lead to improvement or remission of the illness[35].

CHAPTER ELEVEN THIRD EPISODE – PART 2 MY BATTLE WITH OCD

As if my manic attack wasn't bad enough, I also developed an increased tendency toward obsessive-compulsive disorder (OCD) behavior. I had read that an obsession is an uncontrollable thought or fear that causes duress. A compulsion is a ritual or action that someone often repeats. Symptoms of OCD can be triggered by a mental health condition such as bipolar disorder. I felt certain I had this malady.

I had an extreme need for order, and began to feel stressed when objects were out of place. When I organized cans or bottles on my pantry shelves, they always had to be stacked with their front labels facing forward. Cans of tuna fish needed to have each of these labels perfectly aligned with one another before I was satisfied. Bottles were situated from shortest to tallest. None of the objects could touch any of their neighbors. They were like soldiers standing at attention.

The same obsessive-compulsive behavior still applies to objects in my house: bottles of shampoo, shaving cream, and deodorant—all must have their labels facing outward before I can leave the house. Paintings and other wall hangings must be hung with precision.

Another unraveling compulsion is to check repeatedly to ensure my kitchen appliances are turned off and the door is locked before bedtime . . . and then to get out of bed and check a second time just in case. Once, during a bipolar episode, I mistakenly skipped my ritual of checking all the lights before leaving my house. When I returned home, the basement light was on. I felt certain there was a burglar in the house. I called my sister, Katy, who assured me it wasn't necessary to dial 9-1-1. Instead, she stayed on the telephone with me until I checked downstairs and determined there were no strangers on the premises.

I still always bless myself once in the sign of the cross before driving anywhere. When I leave home for an extended vacation, I find it impossible to exit the front door until I've touched all my Archie Manning framed photographs. This is to guarantee good luck on my journey. During my tennis days, I would click my heels once in between points before I was ready to resume play.

I am convinced that the numbers 1:11 and 11:11 on a digital clock are a sign that something positive is about to happen. They always seem to appear when I randomly glance at my watch around those times of day. I'll remain fixated on the numbers until they eventually switch to 1:12 or 11:12, and I can continue where I was before the interruption.

Despite my obvious OCD behavior over the years, there is still a method to my madness concerning my suits and other dress clothes. While to the casual eye they may appear to be strewn in disarray, they are actually carefully placed over furniture to remain wrinkle-free.

My Father's Death

My father died in April 2003 from a heart ailment we had known about for years. Tests showed three arteries were one hundred percent blocked and the fourth seventy-five percent clogged. He had undergone quadruple bypass surgery and, in 1996, had a defibrillator installed to maintain his heartbeat.

It was emotionally painful to witness someone who was once a powerful man slowly diminish into frailty from 1996 over the next seven years until 2003. His feet had swollen and were tightly wrapped with bandages to improve circulation. Ironically, the last time he was able to walk was in January at a memorial service commemorating the twenty-year anniversary of our brother Jon's passing at the age of thirty-four.

My brother-in-law helped to physically support my father as he stumbled his way toward his pew at the memorial service he had vowed to attend. I was too much in the throes of an oncoming bipolar episode to be of much assistance.

During the next three months, my father experienced a slow and sometimes agonizing death, as his body functions deteriorated. One night near the end, his defibrillator failed, and our family gathered at his hospital bed preparing for the worst.

I drove the late night twenty-mile distance from my home to the hospital with my sister, Marlene following in her car. Along the way, a police officer pulled me over for erratic driving and unintentionally running a red light. My sister gestured for the officer to approach her vehicle and explained the situation. He promptly escorted us to the emergency room at the hospital. We joined our other siblings who were already on the scene, as my father drifted in and out of consciousness. I was prepared to say goodbye.

At one point when he stirred, I prodded him, "Dad, who's your favorite football team?"

"The Cleveland Browns," he immediately responded as we all shared a chuckle. Thankfully, he survived that scare, and joyfully lived to see another day.

About three weeks later, my father experienced his final coherent moment while sitting up in his same hospital bed with our family gathered around him. We all laughed and reminisced, and he made the proclamation, "Someday, we're all going to be together again in heaven."

Although some of my siblings may have inwardly scoffed at this suggestion, it was neither the time nor the place to ruin this rare family moment.

At that juncture, we took turns dropping by to visit. As luck would have it, I was the last family member to see him alive. By then he was thrashing in his bed as a nurse unmercifully crammed barely edible food into his mouth.

Eyes closed, my father shouted, "I want to die!"

After the nurse left his room, I hovered over his bed where he now lay peacefully. I stared at his face and observed his lips slowly turning blue. I shook him several times and mumbled, "Dad, please don't die," as my eyes welled up with tears.

Color returned to his face momentarily.

I leaned over and kissed him on his forehead and said, "Dad, you're the greatest father in the world." As the words left my mouth, I wondered to myself almost angrily why I had lied to him as he stared death in the face. Was it because I suddenly felt pity for someone who had caused me so much pain and scarred my self-confidence forever? I had been unfairly deprived of a childhood role model and now he was about to disappear forever. I struggled for an explanation to account for my compassionate sentiment. I was only able to suggest one word:

Forgiveness.

At the funeral parlor two days later, I received permission to play a song for him as a final farewell tribute. It was a song that he and I had co-written when he was hosting the fiftieth reunion of WWII with his army buddies at his home in the Poconos. It had been a real father and son bonding moment, and I wanted to relive it one last time before they closed his casket.

While playing the CD, it began to skip, and I had to shut it off. I removed it from the CD player and flung it across the room like a Frisbee. I broke down in tears in a bipolar-induced moment. One of my family members, who was aware of my mental instability, hurried over to console me.

In the cemetery after the funeral, I was given a folded United States banner that is awarded to all veterans of war upon their death. My father had instructed that he wanted me to keep it. I still have it on display in my living room as a constant reminder of my bittersweet relationship with my dad.

At the Recording Studio

Shortly after my father's death, I called my new doctor late one night and left an urgent message on his answering machine. I frantically told him I was scared concerning my new mood stabilizer, and I was going to switch back to my original medication. But by now I sensed it was too late. The irreversible damage had been done. This would be the start of my third and worst episode.

It was after midnight and I still had enough control of my senses to realize I wasn't going to make my scheduled session at the recording studio the following night. I figured I should let them know. I called Dan and groggily left him a barely coherent, cryptic message. At the end of my message, I said something along the lines of, "Dan, it's been nice knowing you . . . I just called to say goodbye."

As it turned out, I did wind up seeing Dan one last time at the studio before my episode became full-blown, just not the following evening there. He immediately confronted me while standing near the mixing board, "I think you're starting to lose it again."

He referenced the frightening voice mail I had left and inquired if I wanted him to play it back. Apparently, he hadn't erased it.

"No. I'd rather you didn't."

I considered Dan a good friend and more than just a business associate. It meant a lot to me that he was concerned about my welfare. I just wished he didn't think of me as someone who had gone crazy after a friendship spanning twenty years.

It frustrated me that no one seemed to have a handle on my mental illness. It convinced me I had an obligation to educate people on my bipolar condition. In part, that's what I hope sharing my personal story does.

Listen up, everybody: I do not have demons, I am not drunk, I am not neurotic, I am not drugged, I am not crazy, and I certainly do not have a brain tumor (at least, I hope not). I have bipolar disorder, formerly known as manic-depression.

June 27, 2003

Back at the manufacturing firm where I worked, I was one of the last people in the office on an ominous evening that marked the heightening of episode three. As I sat with my eyes glued to the computer, a coworker repeatedly passed by, retrieving copies of sales invoices from the printer.

"Steve, you look bleary-eyed. Go home for crying out loud!"

What he didn't realize was that I was trying to get out of there and go home, but there was one slight problem. I couldn't figure out how to shut down my computer. My mental condition had made me so worn-out, I was unable to concentrate on completing this simple task.

I clicked on the shutdown menu. There was a dropdown menu with a selection of choices, including logoff and restart. Instead of simply hitting logoff, I continued to restart the computer.

I couldn't comprehend why my frigging computer wouldn't shut off! No exaggeration, I must have sat there for a half hour caught up in this futile effort. Finally, I heeded my coworker's advice and simply left the computer on. Obviously, it was not the preferred choice to abandon it, but it was either that or throw it out the flipping window. Surely, our IT department would be sympathetic to my situation.

I didn't know it then, but I would not return to the office for some time. My father's recent passing had taken a toll on my fragile state of mind. Once more, my car drove itself home.

CLINICAL OVERVIEW (CHAPTER ELEVEN)

*H*ow *can a person diagnosed with bipolar disorder best cope with this mental illness?*

Bipolar disorder (BD) is an illness and, like other incurable illnesses, its symptoms must be managed. For a person living with bipolar disorder this often means:

- Education about bipolar disorder
- Bipolar disorder therapy
- Learning ways of coping with bipolar symptoms and life stress
- Medication treatment
- A regimented daily schedule including good sleep, hygiene, eating and exercising

These factors can affect almost every moment of the day and put a lot of pressure on those living with bipolar. But these steps are necessary to try to prevent future bipolar episodes.

Side effects from bipolar medication treatment can also create additional pressures on the patient. Living with bipolar disorder often means living with an array of side effects such as:

- Fatigue
- Nausea
- Battles with weight

- Headaches
- And others that are specific to the person

Side effects can make a person feel physically as well as mentally sick, leading to missed days of work or school or not being able to fully take part in family activities.

The key to successfully living with bipolar is to stick strictly to the bipolar treatment plan, get early medical intervention for any occurring episodes, and to reach out to others for support and help when needed.

Living with someone with bipolar is not easy either. The loved one must support someone with an incurable illness, which often places extreme stress on the relationship. Clear boundaries need to be drawn between what a loved one can or cannot do for the person with BD. Living with a bipolar spouse often harms the mental health of the loved one, making the relationship even more challenging.

When living with someone with BD, it's important to remember:

- The illness is not your or your loved one's fault. You cannot "fix" the bipolar but you can support the person with bipolar. Don't ever tell them to just "snap out of it."
- Each person experiences bipolar disorder differently, so while education is crucial, listening to the loved one with bipolar is equally important.
- You can offer to help with health care appointments, medication schedules and the like, but you shouldn't become the "bipolar drill sergeant."
- It takes time for treatment to work and it may be many months before your loved one is stable. Patience and support is crucial during this time[36].

When living with a bipolar person, it's also important to get help for you, too. Agencies like the National Alliance on Mental Illness[37] and the Depression and Bipolar Support Alliance[38] are useful in connecting with other loved ones living with a person with bipolar disorder.

Family therapy for the person living with bipolar and their loved ones is also a good way of handling the stresses of a mental illness.

CHAPTER TWELVE THIRD EPISODE – PART 3 TROUBLE WITH THE LAW

I don't remember everything about this unfortunate incident, but I've pieced a lot together from my own memories and details provided by my neighbors Carol, Shaun, Peg, and Mark, who were present when it happened. My sisters Marlene, and Linda were also aware of the situation. On Saturday, June 28, 2003, the local police were dispatched to my residence.

To back up a bit, I returned from work on the evening of Friday, June 27 around 6:30 p.m. I was extremely disoriented and barely able to drive home from the office. I parked my car incorrectly in my next-door neighbor's driveway. Since Mark was new to the block, we had not yet met.

Later, Mark said he arrived home around 1:30 a.m. on Saturday and discovered my car in his driveway. I stood in my doorway, dazed and confused. Earlier, I'd tried to fit my house key into the lock on his door to gain entry to the home I had mistakenly thought was mine. I had since spent the entire seven hours outside my place primarily attempting to access Mark's townhouse, thinking I resided there. I wasn't trying to break in or do anything illegal or harmful. I was simply disoriented as I approached Mark and asked for his assistance.

Mark called 9-1-1 after he opened his garage door, and I wandered in, thinking he was helping me access my own home, after complaining to him I could not get my garage door opener to work right. I became further confused when I walked into the house and upstairs to use the bathroom. I finally realized, as I saw the orange furniture in the living room that I was in the wrong place. I sat down on the unfamiliar couch and apparently tried to use his remote control for the television.

Three police officers in two patrol cars responded at about 2:00 a.m. In my stupor, I inadvertently locked Mark out of his own townhouse via the garage. He and the police entered through the front door. Although Mark was understandably flustered by the whole chain of events, I remained very calm and docile throughout the entire incident. As a result, he did not fear I was harmful in any way.

"Would you like to press charges for trespassing?" the police gruffly inquired.

"No, I'm fine . . . just please don't ticket my car for being left on the street."

The police decided it was best to simply leave my car in Mark's driveway for the night.

"He appears to be drugged or overmedicated," Mark said worriedly. "Are you sure you don't want us to take him in?"

"No, I don't feel threatened by him."

The police were able to find my true address on my driver's license. Two of the officers walked the two doors down to my residence. For some reason, they began banging repeatedly on my front door to see if I was home, even though they'd just encountered me at my neighbor's house, and I had only minutes earlier willingly handed them my driver's license.

The loud and unwarranted knocking awakened another neighbor, Peg, inciting her dog to bark repeatedly. She got out of bed and approached the police officers.

"Can I ask what the matter is?"

"Yes, ma'am, do you know who Steve West is?"

Peg was baffled since they were reading my name directly from my driver's license. I was still sitting at Mark's place with him and the other police officer. Even so, one of the other police officers continued to bang on my door to see if I might be home.

"He looks like he's drunk. I think we're going to take him to police headquarters."

"No, officer, please. He's a very nice guy," Peg said.

She remained confused when the officer persisted in pounding on my front door and then instructed her to leave the scene. The only reason I was not arrested was because Mark refused to press charges. The night ended with the police eventually escorting me back to my house. They assisted me in opening my front door with the house key I had been carrying all along.

A third neighbor from across the street overhead the officers talking to me as they walked me inside my house, "Does everything look okay?" they asked.

I groggily responded. "Yes."

The police left my residence and the 9-1-1 escapade concluded around 2:45 a.m.

***

Later that morning at around 9:00 a.m., my next-door neighbor, Carol noticed me sitting in my parked car in the wrong driveway. I vaguely recall having re-entered my vehicle at some point after 6:00

a.m. I was still dressed in my suit clothes from the night before. Carol could tell I was disoriented, having known me for over five years. She knew I did not drink excessively, but she was also unaware at the time that I suffered from mental illness.

"Move over to the passenger seat," she instructed, sliding into the driver's side.

I quietly complied. She proceeded to pull my car into my driveway. Walking me to my house, she opened the garage door to allow me access. According to Carol, this whole process took about twenty minutes.

At 9:20 a.m., she contacted my sister, Linda, to tell her what was going on. My sister informed her of my bipolar disorder. Carol had followed me up to my bedroom along with her husband, Shaun.

"Where is he now?" inquired my sister.

"Well," said Carol, "the good news, I suppose, is that he appears to at least be temporarily safe. He's sprawled out on his own bed upstairs."

"We need to get him to a hospital for psychiatric treatment right away. This is his third episode."

I suddenly began to choke and cough severely. Carol instructed Shaun to call 9-1-1. My choking fit stopped, so they notified the 9-1-1 operator to cancel their response. They decided to have one of my family members take me to the hospital, since they thought my situation was no longer an emergency. The time was 10:15 a.m.

"The ambulance is already on the way, sir," said the 9-1-1 operator.

Carol and Shaun were surprised when the police responded first at 10:30 a.m.

"He only needs medical treatment," said Carol.

"We're just following policy, ma'am," said the officer.

Carol trailed the two officers inside my house as they marched their way up to my second-floor bedroom. They discovered me lying flat on my bed in a semi-conscious state. Once again, as they had misdiagnosed the night before, they assumed I was drunk.

It was early in the morning on a Saturday, and I was lying peacefully in the comfort of my own bedroom and yet they thought I was drunk. There was no smell of alcohol on my breath. It was around thirty minutes since Carol had last spoken to Linda. She was now talking with her again to update her on the situation. The ambulance had arrived and was waiting downstairs.

I vaguely recall Carol putting the cordless telephone next to my ear. "Do you want to speak with your sister, Linda?"

"No," I declined in my weakened state.

According to Carol, I began to wail, "I don't want to go to the bad place." This was meant as a reference to hell, though Carol later told me she assumed I was afraid of the psychiatric unit.

Carol handed the cordless telephone to one of the officers.

"My brother is on medications," said my sister. "I think they're in his kitchen cabinets downstairs. He's suffering from a mental illness."

The officer followed my sister's instructions and found my meds downstairs. He even brought them later to the hospital. The officers were now clearly aware of my mental instability, and the cause of my erratic behavior. At this point, I should have been transported by the EMS workers to the psychiatric unit of the nearby hospital.

Instead, Carol witnessed the officers interrogate me. She told me that they became irate when I would not answer their questions.

"What's going on?" they demanded.

Apparently, they thought I was deliberately being difficult and unresponsive. They had already been informed about my medical condition, so what were they still doing in my bedroom? They continued to rattle me with basic inquiries such as "Do you know what day of the week it is?"

"Saturday," I correctly replied.

Carol said their line of questioning wasted time since they should have been taking me to the hospital.

Instead, one of them lifted my arm up over my forehead.

"Let's see if he lets it drop down on him."

I was able to catch it before it landed on my face.

"He's messing with us," the other officer mumbled.

They turned around and saw Carol still standing on my second-floor landing, observing what was taking place.

He motioned to her. "Please leave the house, ma'am." She reluctantly complied with this order.

It was around this time I began to fully awaken and sat up in bed. Becoming coherent, I saw them standing directly over me. I was both startled and upset.

"What the hell is going on here? Get the fuck out of my bedroom!"

What I perceived as a legitimate reaction, they interpreted as belligerence. I'm sure the police report will reflect I lunged at one of the officers and took a swing at him. This prompted a subsequent criminal charge of aggravated assault on a police officer. The charge was later reduced to simple assault, which is a felony.

However, my version of the story is quite different. After my remarks, I recall the two officers lifting me off the bed and forcefully pressing my body against the headboard. One of them grabbed my left arm, pinned it behind my back, and slapped on a handcuff. The second officer grabbed my right arm, extended it backwards, and roughly applied the other handcuff.

While being cuffed, my arm knocked over the lamp perched on my nightstand. During this process, my right arm and elbow also inadvertently banged into one of the officer's shoulders.

That's my side of the story. I don't care how crazed I may have been at the time, I would never consider hitting an officer of the law, especially when there were two of them and only one of me. They were twice my size and carrying guns. There were no witnesses.

At the Hospital June 28, 2003

Shortly after this transpired, the police notified my sister, Marlene, that I had been arrested. She was understandably shocked and angry at this dramatic twist of events. The officers had already had me transported to the local hospital for evaluation. I don't recall being read my rights or informed as to what my charges were.

Marlene contacted the hospital by telephone and spoke to the head nurse concerning my need for psychiatric treatment. She emphasized I had already experienced two prior hospital stays due to this illness.

"I'm sorry," said the nurse, "we can only conduct a physical examination here to determine whether he should be sent to the psychiatric unit at our other facility for further evaluation."

When I was first unceremoniously delivered to the hospital, I woke up strapped to a bed, flat on my back. My wrist restraints were secured so tightly I had lost all circulation in my hands.

"Please loosen my straps. My hands are turning purple!"

The nurse replied in a genuinely sympathetic voice, "I'm sorry, but I'm not allowed to."

Then she approached my mid-section, holding some device in her hand. It turns out it was a catheter. She inserted it into my penis. I had never experienced this pain before, and I had been taken by surprise.

"Owwwww!" I shrieked in agony, jolting up in bed, except I was restrained from moving too far.

I experienced an image in my head that I was Jesus Christ being crucified on the cross. My hands were strapped so tightly, they felt as if they were nailed to the bed boards.

"Please, nurse, please give me something . . . anything to take away the pain!"

This time, she obliged. She apparently had permission to inject me with a needle. I was asleep within seconds.

Before I nodded off, I heard the two police officers who were standing about ten feet behind me. They were apparently watching a rerun of Seinfeld on television and chuckling while I suffered mercilessly. I conjured up a vision of them being forced to experience an episode of unbearable torment for the rest of eternity based on their inhumane treatment of me in my vulnerable state.

Meanwhile, as I lay there unconscious, my sister was still on the telephone with the stubborn nurse, attempting to get me psychiatric treatment.

The nurse responded, "The alternative may be sending him to the county jail for treatment since he was arrested."

"You don't seem to understand the serious negative impact it will have on his condition if he isn't treated immediately," my sister screamed.

"Miss, please calm down, and stop shouting at me. I'm just following protocol."

"I'd like to speak to the treating doctor right away," Marlene said.

"I'm sorry, miss, he's not available."

My sister hung up the telephone and called back thirty minutes later. She was informed I had been removed to the county jail because of my arrest. Strange as it seems, apparently their policy was to send me to jail where I would receive further evaluation.

Marlene called the police officers who had taken me to the correctional facility. "What can I do to get my brother released?" she asked in an increasingly frantic voice.

They seemed docile and were now obviously aware of my medical condition since my charges had been reduced. It was sometime in the afternoon on Saturday.

"After getting to know your brother today, he seems like a nice guy," one of the officers said.

"Can I speak to him?" she pleaded over the phone.

"We're sorry. ma'am, but you're not allowed to speak to anyone at the county jail, including the doctor there."

They added that no visitors were even allowed until Monday. Today was Saturday. She could not post bail until Tuesday. My bail was set at one hundred thousand dollars.

"Are you at least giving him his medications?" she inquired in desperation.

"We're sorry, ma'am, but we can't disclose that information."

As it turned out, it wouldn't be until Monday night she could bring me my proper medications and request they be administered to me.

Four days in County Jail July, 2003

It had been later in the day on Saturday when I was taken by the two police officers to the county jail where I spent the next four days. The two officers who escorted me were now being much nicer. I suspected this was because they realized that I had family members who cared about me. This time I was handcuffed with my hands in front of me, and less tightly, to minimize pain.

At the facility, the police officers removed my handcuffs. Once they left the building, new police officers proceeded to abuse me verbally, rob me, and humiliate me as will be illustrated in the ensuing hours.

I was left alone with the officer in charge. He had an intimidating physique, and a mean-spirited demeanor that frightened me almost as much as the loaded gun he carried in his holster. I didn't know what to expect since I had never been in jail before. My bipolar episode was still in full swing and beyond my control, because I had been declined treatment in their normal psychiatric unit since my arrest.

Instead, I was set to receive a medical evaluation and monitoring at the county jail. Meanwhile, I had already missed a day of my medications, which included mood stabilizers and ones that addressed paranoia. My current stabilizing pills (which I was recently switched to because it promoted weight loss), were apparently ineffective, and had led to my current situation.

There was no doubt in my mind, even in my crazed state, that I needed to switch back to my previous medication. This would be later confirmed by my doctors. I was also denied two other medications to treat depression while in jail.

The officer in charge inquired of me in a gruff voice. "Why were you sent here?"

"I suffer from bipolar disorder."

Before I could elaborate, he interjected, "Gotcha, so you're one of them bipolars."

After recording some background information on me, he proceeded to fingerprint me *eleven* times to acquire a total of seven sets of prints for each hand. This included the difficult side of my pinky. Nine of these sets were taken with red ink.

When I supposedly messed up on the first set of prints, although they appeared fine to me, he wisecracked, "West, you're starting to piss me off already."

On three occasions during this laborious process, he had me literally sprint to the bathroom sink across the room to clean my hands and remove the red ink. Since I was deep in the grips of a bipolar episode, my hands were spasmodic at times. This only initiated additional verbal abuse on his part.

"West, I've had a lot of bipolars in here, but you're the dumbest."

These constant derogatory remarks only served to make me more flustered. After what seemed like an eternity, he finally secured what he considered to be six sets of acceptable fingerprints. He then required one additional set on the computer.

When he claimed the initial one was not okay, I asked him innocently, "How can a computer make a mistake? I used to work for a major software company."

He lightened up momentarily and said the second set of prints taken on the computer was fine. We were finally finished with this exasperating process, but my hell was just beginning.

I was next escorted into a much smaller room where I was ordered to strip naked in front of another male officer. The officer in charge instructed me, "Grab your balls three times and lift them up in the air where I can see them."

I couldn't believe this was taking place, but I did as I was told. He then ordered me in a stern voice, "Now turn around and face the wall with your arms and legs spread-eagled against it."

I was terrified as to what might happen next and, sure enough, my humiliation was not finished yet.

"Crouch down and then back up again."

Please, God, let this be over, I prayed. Fortunately, my prayers were answered. There would be no physical abuse like the kind I had read about that apparently occurs often in jails.

Obviously, this whole process was both unnecessary and severely degrading. This was a very crude and perverted form of being strip searched, if that's what it was about in the first place. The other officers had already determined I was not armed with any weapons. I had been handcuffed the whole time while under their earlier supervision.

Now I was stark naked while the two officers at me throughout this sadistic process. Maybe I was naïve, but I couldn't believe this cruel behavior was tolerated inside jails or correctional facilities.

I had been under the mistaken impression that minor offenses were treated with a mild and short-term incarceration. Instead I met many other inmates while I was locked up, perhaps ten or more, that were in for extremely minor crimes. Some of them confided they were receiving horrible treatment as well.

One inmate told me he had been in jail for over a year. "I have no family members or friends who could post bail. My criminal offense was jaywalking."

Another informed me, "My crime was being caught double-parking at a meter while I ran inside a convenience store to buy a pack of cigarettes."

He was behind bars on a long-term basis for lack of a quarter. Some of the inmates told me, "Nobody even knows I'm in here."

I have since vowed to myself that if ever given the opportunity down the road to help these forgotten souls, I will try my best to do so.

We were continually under surveillance by armed guards. At one point, I heard someone getting roughed up by multiple police officers and dragged down the hall. He was called a troublemaker.

The next step in my ordeal after my perverted "strip-search" was being told to take a one-minute, cold shower in a stall. Upon completion, I was ordered to turn my socks inside out before I put them back on. Other than my underwear, they kept my clothes. The officer in charge instructed me to don a pair of gray overalls. I struggled to do so in my run-down mental state.

When I accidentally put them on backwards, he called me stupid. I was handed oversized bright orange shoes and informed I was now an inmate.

He ordered me to remove my wallet from my pants pocket. I had still been dressed in my suit from the previous Friday, my last day at work. When I handed it to him, he tossed it on a table and scattered my credit cards. It had recently been payday and my wallet contained two hundred and forty dollars in twenty-dollar bills. This money was never returned to me. It was not even mentioned on my *Inmate Property Form* when my stay was eventually over.

Along with the other inmates, I was fed slop to eat, and was eventually allowed to see the tending doctor. He appeared to be unaware of my medications. I wasn't informed my sisters were present until I was finally permitted to meet with them. We conversed through a glass partition as I struggled in my severely paranoid state of mind.

"We want you to take your medications," they insisted, practically begging me. I was confused if I should trust them. Was their advice beneficial to my overall welfare?

It was already Monday. Where had the time gone? I had inconceivably not taken my medications since Thursday night. Marlene peered at me through a booth window at the jail. It was apparent my condition was rapidly deteriorating. My paranoia had become so advanced that I refused to see her or the rest of my family. She was finally able to post bail and have me released at 5:00 p.m. on Tuesday.

Marlene later informed me that she and Linda had visited me on another occasion; but I was so traumatized I was unsure if they were really there. Marlene had asked the staff if she could poke her head around to assure me she was there. Her request was denied since it was supposedly against regulations.

It had been four days of hell since I had been admitted to jail, and I was now being released. But, I didn't go quietly. I saw several armed guards sternly approaching me.

"They're coming to get me!" I wailed in terror.

They instructed me to remove my overalls, so I could put my suit clothes back on. When I took off my overalls I wasn't wearing any underwear, and I began running naked down the corridor with the guards in fast pursuit. I was able to elude their slippery grasps until, finally, they managed to corral and dress me. They had to restrain me as I refused to cooperate. After the medical staff gave me a sedative injection, I was roughly placed in handcuffs behind my back by the guards and loaded into the back of a police van. This rugged treatment was needed to ensure no further drama on my part. It may have also been necessitated because of my spinning in circles and snapping my fingers in the air. I was officially out of my mind.

***

The following is a summary of expenses, claims and losses from this entire unfortunate episode. I kept a partial diary of many of the events immediately after I returned home, which is why some of them are so fresh in my mind fifteen years later.

- Thirty work days at sixty percent of pay due to prolonged disability: $1,730.
- An additional twenty days for outpatient treatment at a cost of one hundred forty dollars per week: $560.
- A sixty dollar daily copay for my eighteen day stay at the institution: $1,080.
- My confiscated money at jail that was never replaced: $240.
- Attorney's fee and court costs: $1,000.
- The hospital sent me approximately $170,000 in medical bills. The ambulance charge alone was $19,000. Insurance will only cover customary expenses. Anticipated debt: $35,000.
- Punitive damages for pain and suffering at the hands of the police during my arrest at my house and upon my stay at the correctional facility where I was verbally abused.
- Estimated out-of-pocket expenses: $40,000.

CLINICAL OVERVIEW (CHAPTER TWELVE)

W*hy is it critical to educate police concerning the signs of mental illnesses such as bipolar disorder?*
At a time of heightened concern over police shootings, a 2016 report estimates that people with mental illness are sixteen times more likely than others to be killed in confrontations with law officers.

Approximately one in four fatal police encounters involve someone with mental disorders, according to a report released by the Virginia-based Treatment Advocacy Center, which focuses on the needs of people with grave mental illness.

"The problem stems from a lack of police training, as well as a lack of treatment for those with serious mental illness," said John Snook, the report's coauthor and executive director of the Treatment Advocacy Center. "In many cases, people with serious mental illness do not get treatment until their behavior attracts the attention of the police.[39]"

"If this were any other medical condition, people would be up in arms," Snook said. "What we need to do is treat the person before the police are ever called. This is a mental illness, but we respond by calling the police and arresting a person."

According to the report, nearly eight million Americans suffer from a serious mental condition that "disorders their thinking," such as schizophrenia or bipolar disorder. On any given day, half these patients are not taking medications or receiving other care.

"Police are being forced to be mental health counselors without training," said Jim Pasco, executive director of the National Fraternal Order of Police, the largest police organization in the country. "It underscores a real tragedy: the total collapse of the mental health system in the United States. People who should be wards of the hospital are wards of the street."

"People with mental illness are no more violent than others," Snook said. "But without treatment, they often end up homeless or arrested for relatively minor offenses, such as loitering, shoplifting or urinating in public."

Some law office departments have formed crisis intervention teams, whose members have special training in dealing with mental disorders. Training focuses on ways to calm people during a breakdown, rather than using force.

A 2016 article on the website of Psychiatry Online[40] discussed contact between police and people with mental disorders. Eighty-five unique studies covering 329,461 cases that met the criteria were investigated. Data reported in twenty-one studies indicated that twenty-five percent of people with mental disorders have been arrested. Data reported in thirteen studies suggest that one percent of police encounters involve people with mental disorders.

A prevailing sentiment is that many of these interactions are undesirable, unnecessary, and avoidable. By providing estimates regarding the rates of contact between police and people with mental disorders, this study illuminates the magnitude of the issue and supplies an empirically supported reference point to scholars and practitioners in this area.

CHAPTER THIRTEEN THIRD EPISODE – PART 4 PSYCHIATRIC WARD

T he next thing I remember is waking up at the institution. Many of my recollections there are understandably blurred as I was drifting in and out of mental coherency. I had finally been delivered to a professional psychiatric unit for treatment. In retrospect, I question if my illness was diagnosed and addressed properly. My condition didn't stabilize, but continued to worsen dramatically during my thirteen-day stay.

I was diagnosed psychotic, disorganized, paranoid, and not likely to improve without aggressive treatment, which included medications.

One of the staff mentioned I had three *nervous breakdowns* over a period of eight years. This indicated they may have mistaken my bipolar disorder for another malady. It made me curious as to why they didn't have accurate records for me. I wasn't sure if a family member was present at my time of admission to clarify matters.

My extended stay at the hospital was eventful. I don't remember much, but I've pieced it together from a variety of sources such as eyewitnesses, discharge summaries and comprehensive hospital records.

During the initial screening, I declined to answer most of the questions. I refused to get up and get dressed.

As the doctor interviewed me, I kept my head down. Occasionally I would scream, "God, Oh God." Other times, I simply held my head in my hands and said nothing.

Unexpectedly, I looked up and asked: "Can I have some snacks and a drink?"

"Would you like to come to the dining room and get some there?" The doctor asked.

"No, I changed my mind. I am excusing you . . . you can leave."

Sensing my unwillingness to cooperate, he decided that it was fruitless to continue our conversation, so he left. Once again, I was left alone with just my delusional thoughts.

***

The following morning, without any provocation, I threw a carton of milk at another patient. I was preoccupied, lost deep in my hallucinations and hearing voices. Only this time, they weren't the voices of Sonya, Cliff, or Priscilla. I believed they were coming directly from God. The good news is that I wasn't suicidal. The bad news was I needed to be placed in solitary observation.

During my stay in the psychiatric ward, I did not attend many groups. I was exhibiting unprovoked, angry outbursts. I suspect it was because I was being treated with incorrect mood stabilizers. One of these meds had triggered my third episode in the first place.

The agonizing voices refused to stop haunting me. During one of my daily visits with the psychiatrist, I hesitated to reveal what the voices were telling me. Finally, I raised myself off the bed in a standing position and stared at the door. "Jesus Christ saved me," I proclaimed matter-of-factly.

Later, while attending one of my rare group sessions, I announced, "I want to leave here as soon as possible and return to work."

I demonstrated little insight into my own condition. This was evident the following night in the dining room when I slapped another patient, again without provocation.

"Give me a gun and let me shoot him in the head," I shouted angrily.

I was placed in seclusion in the Quiet Room to distance myself from the other patients until I calmed down. This is a restricted area for patients with advanced mental illness who have exhibited violent behavior. The staff determined that I did not require restraints or a locked door at this time even though I had physically assaulted someone. I'm unsure why. Maybe because it was my first offense. I soon fell asleep and was snoring loudly. Later in the day, during therapy, I still displayed paranoia. The voices had returned: God told me that someone was bad.

I must have maintained at least some semblance of sanity because I was able to communicate to my doctor the need to return to my original medications. This entire episode had transpired because of changing my medication simply because it promoted weight loss.

On one particularly stressful night that would have been comical given any other circumstances, Marlene, her companion, and my niece came to visit. They witnessed me lying on the floor like an overturned turtle screaming: "Heineken! Heineken! Heineken!"

Marlene grasped me by one hand, and her friend lifted me up by the other and walked me back and forth across the hall. Her friend began to cry.

"Mom," said my niece, "Is Uncle Steve going to be all right?"

"Yes, honey, he's going to be fine."

As my stay continued, I notified the staff if I was feeling tired. They observed I was still exhibiting paranoia about some of the other patients. I constantly stared at people as if I were going to attack them. One morning I even threatened a female staff member. I entered the rooms of several patients but couldn't explain why. It wasn't with the intent to harm anyone.

This eventually took a dramatic turn for the worse. While watching television with the group one evening, I began directing hostile remarks at my peers. When confronted by the other patients, I apologized to everyone and continued watching television. The staff came to investigate the matter after the initial commotion. As soon as they left, I proceeded to physically assault an innocent elderly patient. I grabbed his cane.

Witnesses stated that I growled, "Give me that! You're the Devil. I'm going to kill you!" Add that man to the growing list of people I had threatened to kill during my odyssey. I struck him on his right wrist and over the head several times. Fortunately, he didn't suffer any fractures, though he did need to wear a support on his wrist and complained of headaches after the incident.

The Quiet Room in Restraints

Because of that threat to kill someone, on July 13, 2003, I was placed in the Quiet Room in restraints. I was continuously monitored on a one-to-one level of observation.

While strapped down, I was often agitated and restless. At one point I began pulling at the restraints and cursing. However, after over two hours, my behavior expectation had been met. I was rational and cooperative, so my straps were removed.

Before I was released from the Quiet Room, I was administered the following post restraint patient briefing:

"Do you know why you were in restraints?" The doctor asked.

"No," I calmly replied.

"Did being in restraints help you gain control of yourself?"

"Yes."

"Did you feel safe while you were in restraints?"

"Yes."

"Did you feel your privacy respected?"

"Yes."

"Were you given a chance to gain control of yourself before you were put in restraints?"

"No."

"Did you ask for medication when you started to feel out of control?"

"No."

"What could you have done differently to stay out of restraints?"

I remained silent.

"What can we do to help you avoid restraint in the future?"

Once again, I said nothing.

An attendant escorted me back to my room. There I spent the remainder of the night under the watchful eye of a hall monitor situated outside my door. Understandably, a decision was made to transfer me to a more advanced institution because the other patients were becoming frightened of me. The next day, I was transported to the psychiatric ward of a second hospital via ambulance on a stretcher and in restraints. The new facility was equipped for better treatment. My journey was just beginning.

The Second Hospital The Quiet Room (Revisited)

It was at the new psychiatric ward that I ultimately began receiving life-saving medical attention. During the first ten days, my condition was so severe that my return to sanity was questionable. It was determined that I required constant supervision within the four confined walls of the Quiet Room.

Upon intake, my doctor reported, "The patient was initially extremely confused and psychotic, having multiple auditory hallucinations, paranoid ideation, thoughts of communications from outside sources, hyperactive, flight of ideas and distractible." Those are all descriptive words for bipolar disorder.

The doctor interviewed me to determine my present state of awareness: "Can you name four presidents?"

I answered correctly.

"Do you know what today's date is?"

I replied with the wrong date: "July 26, 2003." It was the 14th.

"Does your employer know about your hospitalization?"

"No. I never called them."

"Do you know why you're here?"

"People are after me. They're trying to eliminate me."

"Are you hearing voices?"

"Yes, voices are controlling me. I've had thoughts of suicide and killing people in the past. I don't feel like hurting anyone or myself now, but I want you to know."

It was after midnight when the questioning stopped and I was taken to the Quiet Room.

July 15, 2003

The staff informed me that I snored very loudly overnight. When I awoke, I heard voices again.

"I'm afraid somebody is going to kill me . . . they're going to poison me. A satellite dish is watching me," I rambled to one of the social workers, Denise.

Apparently, she had been assigned to complete a one-on-one assessment with me in the Quiet Room. I repeated my delusional claim, "There's a satellite dish watching me." I insisted, "They are trying to eliminate me."

"Who is?" she inquired.

"The bad people. I've tried to kill eight people in the past ten years."

My thought process remained disjointed. She asked me if I was hearing voices.

I nodded. "Pretty beautiful girls go to hell." I continued to babble. "I am not Superman. I cannot burst out of here!"

She hurriedly jotted down notes

I stood up and announced. "Good morning, I am God! It was on the paper at the meeting. It was part of the brainwashing."

Later, in our afternoon session, I asked her, "Can you read my thoughts?"

"Do you think I can?"

"I guess you don't have the ability, but both have it . . . the good and the bad. Did you get that?"

"I'm not sure what you mean," Denise said.

"I don't know which one you are, but both the good and the bad collect my thoughts."

Around that time, I became agitated and raised a fist at one of the nurses. I was again placed in seclusion.

Marlene waited patiently in the reception area during my session with Denise. She informed my social worker that she would come back to visit me when I was released from the Quiet Room.

"Ever since our father's death," Marlene said, "he's been paranoid . . . thinking he's next."

I was experiencing multiple auditory hallucinations at five levels, including: Loud thoughts inside my head, communications from outside my head, hearing two-way conversations, reading people's minds, and getting messages from radio and television.

July 16 and 17, 2003

My doctor met with me in the Quiet Room.

I explained, "I threatened to hurt staff and peers to keep them from killing me."

He was able to convince me to take my medications that day, but I told him I would not take them anymore. This was because my original psychiatrist had prescribed them.

I became delusional. "My former doctor has a plan to take over the world," I said. "I'm the only one that can save it. I can read other people's thoughts—that's how I know."

I apologized for believing staff was against me, but I was still afraid that I would harm someone. "Why didn't the other hospital tell you I might hurt someone?"

After a brief respite, I was back in seclusion in the Quiet Room.

I began shouting profanities in a threatening and illogical manner at no one in particular. "You people are telling me who was in the picture . . . couldn't be done. I've been kidnapped . . . people told me they opened the door and I should have gotten out then . . . I will next time."

I became even more agitated, and I yelled for the security officers in a paranoid state and complained. "I'm afraid someone is going to hurt me."

July 18, 2003

I remained in seclusion in fear. "I'm going to be attacked by people outside my door." I felt like I was in prison, suspicious and paranoid. I attempted a daring escape from the Quiet Room, thinking it was a police station. "The staff are officers trying to kill me." I said.

Several attendants grabbed me as I struggled to break free from their powerful grips to race down the hall. I had so much adrenaline, I actually carried the three of them on my back for a few steps. They dragged me forcefully back into the Quiet Room where I returned to my cell.

At this point, my mental capacity had slipped so low that the staff suggested I try Electroconvulsive Therapy (ECT). This is a procedure that sends shockwaves through the brain and is typically used only as a last resort. The doctors tried to determine what my eventual outcome would be without it. My sisters said the family continued to pray for me.

Marlene was told by the medical staff, "We're not sure if we can bring him back."

I rejected the ECT treatment, but did agree to try a new trial drug that was only recently approved by the Food and Drug Administration to address my paranoia.

As the day progressed, I continued to rant and rave. "I've been kidnapped . . . I don't need to be here."

One of the staff offered me juice or water.

"Just hand it over." I ordered.

I remained fearful that someone would hurt me. "When I leave there will be a billion-dollar lawsuit!"

Meanwhile, my sisters continued to insist to the staff, "He's such a nice guy when he's stable. It was that switch to the new drug back in May or June that caused him to be depressed and angry for over a month before his hospitalization."

July 21 and 22, 2003

I slept well in seclusion, but I was still concerned about the doctor who continued to harass me. "He is watching me with a special binocular," I said.

I snore very loudly because of sleep apnea. My understanding is that the apnea is often a common side-effect for people with bipolar disorder. My snoring became a subject of playful humor during my time in the Quiet Room. Brien was the employee who oversaw this secluded area. His nickname for me was *Big Bear.*

One night while I was in solitary confinement, an attendant named Mike was assigned to monitor me. He threatened me after I hollered at him from within my cell. In my unstable condition, I was susceptible to sudden outbursts and would shout obscenities without the slightest provocation.

He strolled over to my cell door and took off the white gloves he was wearing. He remarked in anger, "Steve, you know . . . you've got a big fucking mouth when you're safe inside there. Let's see how tough you are when you're not!" Fortunately, it was at the end of his shift and this confrontation occurred as he was leaving. Nothing further came of it except some jawing back and forth. But I was terrified.

The following evening, I sat in a chair in the Quiet Room open area outside my cell as a reward for good behavior. I was permitted to stay there for two hours. Suddenly, I experienced an audio-visual hallucination of an intruder. It was Mike! He was returning for his night shift and carrying a weapon, which I initially identified as a shovel. I knew he was here to harm me or a fellow patient.

I screamed at the top of my lungs. "Mike! Mike! Please don't hurt me!"

I picked up the chair and raised it over my head, prepared to strike.

"Steve, cut it out!" shouted Mike.

Brien hurried in my direction. "Put down the chair, Big Bear!" he ordered.

"But, Brien, he has a weapon!"

"Put down the fucking chair, Big Bear, and get back into your cell or we're going to have to strap you down!"

"No, no, please, don't strap me down, Brien!"

"Then put down the fucking chair and get back into your cell . . . now!"

I did as I was told and returned to my cell.

I observed the lead doctor crouching on the floor in my cell room. I attempted to kick the hallucination.

Brien ran for assistance. I became fearful when many male attendants entered the Quiet Room to help Brien get control. They grabbed Mike. From inside my cell, I heard what sounded like Mike being dragged into the bathroom where the toilet was repeatedly flushed. They left about fifteen minutes later and I peeked around the corner of my cell.

Was I hallucinating again?

Mike's head had been completely shaved, his full head of dark hair completely gone. Could it be that "Mike" was the intruder or one of the other patients? He was strapped to a table in the open area of the Quiet Room where he remained for hours. Finally, he was released from the facility through a rear door, and I never saw him again.

After I calmed down, I said to my social worker, "I feel better now, but a man with a gun tried to shoot me."

Marlene was notified that I had picked up a chair and was prepared to swing it over my head at one of my hallucinations, an attendant who had a shovel. My version of the account alternated between the weapon being a shovel and a gun. I warned the staff that I had a gun and would start using it. I spent the remainder of this eventful night lying down in the seclusion room with no restraints.

July 23, 2003

Every morning during my stay in the Quiet Room, I sat huddled in a fetal position in the corner of my cell. A doctor with a sinister face and glasses crouched next to me, attempting to interact. He held a clipboard.

Was he trying to diagnose me as crazy? Was he trying to force-feed me my meds? My paranoia skyrocketed. I thought he was the enemy and was trying to hurt me. I thought he was able to read my mind. I begged him in a scared voice, "Please stay away from me!"

Brien's voice, out of sight, was assuring. "Big Bear, he's here to help you."

After the doctor left, I stared at the ceiling. In the upper corners were rounded mirrors, like the ones in department stores that detect shoplifting. I screamed again. "They're spying on me!"

"Big Bear, lie down and get some sleep. I didn't hear you snoring last night."

But I stood erect and pressed my back tightly to the wall to escape the view of the mirrors. I peeked around the corner, still in an upright position, until I realized my efforts at hiding were futile. Finally, I heeded Brien's advice and lay down on my bed and went to sleep.

Later that day, I spoke with my social worker through a screen in the seclusion room. She was pleasantly surprised that I remembered her name.

"Where is this hospital located?" I asked her. "Outside my window looks like where my father was buried. I guess I'll be reported for looking out my window."

Denise promised me she wouldn't tell anyone.

"That chair problem was caused by a man who had come back here because he had lost his job. He had a weapon, a gun, and I had to defend myself." I attempted to justify my actions in a subdued voice.

"These thoughts you have been having are being caused by what is known as paranoid ideation," she explained with a soft and sympathetic tone.

"My hallucinations were caused by my switch in meds—is there any way they can be analyzed? . . . I would like to try the open area again, but I will need items to protect me."

"I'll have to check with the doctor first."

"I'm worried about missing work—I'm afraid of losing my job. I never told them I was in here." I suddenly became rattled.

"Relax. Your sister has been in touch with them. Everything is being taken care of for you," Denise reassured me.

***

My audio hallucinations returned overnight, I had a brief exchange with my old friend, Cliff, the conspiracy theorist. I was in a partial dream state, and he was barely audible among the buzzing of the background noise. "Diet soda causes weight gain, just like that medication you were on."

"What are you talking about?"

"They're putting more sugar in the diet soda than the regular brand."

"Who are 'they'?"

"The government. It's all a conspiracy. They're tricking people into trying to lose weight when it's just the opposite. That's why our country is the most overweight nation."

"Why? What's the purpose?"

"Depopulation . . . don't you get it? Obesity, diabetes, heart attacks . . . the New World Order."

"The New World Order! You mean like . . . the Illuminati?"

"They're in on it, too."

The static in my ears was driving me insane. . . I prayed for it to stop.

"You're crazy!" I had to shut down these imaginary voices. They sounded so real.

"And the flu vaccine causes autism," he persisted.

I had read about this controversy before, but I just wanted to go to sleep now.

"The sky isn't blue. It's all an illusion . . . the same with the ocean."

"Stop it!" I covered my ears.

"But, the actual color of fire *is* blue . . . not red. Check out the pilot light on your stove— the flame is blue. The lake of fire in the Bible is blue."

Thankfully, he abruptly stopped speaking, and it seemed my auditory hallucinations were finally over. Then I visually hallucinated a horrific vision of Jack from the recording studio. His angry face appeared in a fiery inferno as the Devil. It reminded me of the scene from *The Wizard of Oz* when Dorothy and her friends first encountered the mighty wizard. Oz's face was projected on the curtain in a cloud of smoke and flames. I visualized Jack going to hell for eternity.

I next fixated on my younger brother Tim. He and his wife had a newborn daughter. I became certain he was my *older* brother and that he had stolen my baby from me. I wanted her back, or he would be going to hell forever, too.

The only other memory I have of the Quiet Room was lying in the dark one night hearing a pair of loud footsteps echoing down the hall in my direction. It was my sister, Linda, and our mutual friend, Joe. The next and final time I would encounter him would be at my sister's wedding. He passed by briefly and snickered: "I was wondering if I would ever see you again." As things developed, I wound up losing him as a friend because of his lack of empathy towards my mental instability.

CLINICAL OVERVIEW (CHAPTER THIRTEEN)

*W*hat *are the similarities and differences between bipolar disorder and schizophrenia?*

Schizophrenia is a primary psychotic disorder, and bipolar disorder (BD) is a primary mood disorder, but these conditions can overlap. Bipolar disorder and schizophrenia have some aspects in common, but also some differences.

Schizophrenia causes symptoms that are more severe than those of BD. People with schizophrenia experience hallucinations and delusions. Hallucinations involve seeing or hearing things that aren't there. Delusions are beliefs in things that aren't true. People with schizophrenia may also experience disorganized thinking in which they are unable to care for themselves.

BD causes strong shifts in energy, mood, and activity levels. A person with BD will switch between extreme excitement or mania, and depression. These shifts can affect the ability to perform daily activities.

Schizoaffective disorder (SD) can be severe and needs to be monitored closely. Depending on the type of mood disorder diagnosed, depression or BD, people will experience different symptoms. Depressed mood: The person will experience feelings of sadness, emptiness, or worthlessness. Manic behavior/BD: The person will experience feelings of euphoria, racing thoughts, and increased risky behavior.

The exact cause of SD is unknown. A combination of factors may contribute to its development:

- Genetics. It tends to run in families.
- Brain chemistry and structure. Brain function and structure may be different in ways that science is only beginning to understand. Brain scans are helping to advance research in this area.
- Stress. Stressful events such as a death in the family, end of a marriage or loss of a job can trigger symptoms or an onset of the illness.
- Drug use. Psychoactive drugs such as LSD have been linked to the development of schizoaffective disorder.

SD can be difficult to diagnose because it has symptoms of both schizophrenia and either depression or BD. To be diagnosed with SD, a person must have the following symptoms:

- A period during which there is a major mood disorder, either depression or mania that occurs while symptoms of schizophrenia are present.
- Delusions or hallucinations for two or more weeks in the absence of a major mood episode.
- Symptoms that meet criteria for a major mood episode are present for most of the total duration of the illness.
- The abuse of drugs or a medication is not responsible for the symptoms.

SD is treated and managed in multiple ways:

- Medications[41], including mood stabilizers, antipsychotic medications and antidepressants

- Psychotherapy, such as cognitive behavioral therapy or family-focused therapy[42].

To be diagnosed with BD, a person must have experienced at least one episode of mania or hypomania. Mental health care professionals use the *Diagnostic and Statistical Manual of Mental Disorders: DSM-5* to diagnose the "type" of BD a person may be experiencing. To determine what type of BD a person has, mental health care professionals assess the pattern of symptoms and how impaired the person is during their most severe episodes[43].

CHAPTER FOURTEEN THIRD EPISODE – PART 5 THE QUIET ROOM

On or about July 24th, I was finally moved to the wing with the rest of the patients, where I began my long road to recovery. They were all dressed in their street clothes, a sign they were further along in their progress. I was still lumbering around in my pajamas in a dazed state.

As I made my way down the long hall, a patient named Amy offered me encouragement. "We weren't sure if we would ever see you back again. We're going to have to give you the *Most Valuable Player* award." Along my slow walk, a dozen people cheered me on, joining Amy in a chorus of, "MVP! MVP! MVP!" It was a scene that brought tears of joy to my eyes.

"Ask them to give you some street clothes," Amy suggested. "They'll let you out of here quicker if you get out of those pajamas."

So I did. Sure enough, the very next day the nurses equipped me with some long and short-sleeved shirts, sweat pants, socks, and underwear. I'll never forget the bright red, extra-large long-sleeved Sponge Bob Square Pants shirt they gave me.

When Amy saw it she said, "Oh, can I please have it? I'll trade you!"

"Sure. What do you have?"

She offered me a selection of travel-oriented T-shirts, and I chose one depicting all the famous pubs in Ireland. I had some trouble fitting into it because of my weight gain.

Later in my afternoon session with my social worker, I told her about my trepidation surrounding my move to the new unit. "I'm experiencing a whole new collage in my head," I said. "Trying to block the thoughts . . . tremendous backlash . . . rumors have spread . . . people are upset and asking 'what did you say?' . . . my mother wants to fuck me . . . I'm scared . . . so much I can't hear what others are saying . . . This is from the transistor radio at the sleep study, the good guys and the bad guys."

"Our records show you recently had two sleep studies. Is that right?" she asked.

"Yes, can you hear my collection of thoughts?"

"No, I can't."

"I had voices in my head, but now they are thoughts within my mind," I said. This marked day ten of my hospitalization. Now that I was in the non-secluded wing, I noticed a gentleman named Robert stayed near me at all times, but did not seem to be a patient. His room was across the hall from mine, and even when I got up in the middle of the night, he would follow me. I suspect his job was to monitor my safety, especially after what happened with Mike. This added to my comfort level on my road back to a complete recovery. Thankfully, there were no further incidents as my paranoia continued to decrease with each passing day.

I sat with the rest of the group periodically, but I still preferred being alone. One night while watching Seinfeld in the television room, I thought I was another character along with Jerry, Elaine, George and

Kramer. I was convinced their dialogue was directed at me. I laughed and responded to them.

Judging from their good-natured comments, I realized the other patients had noticed my strange behavior. "Steve, it's nice to hear you laugh for a change," they said. "We'd like to see this side of you more often," they added playfully. I began to participate in some of the groups. My favorite class was art therapy, where we had the opportunity to draw pictures describing our feelings. One time, I became angry at another patient for grabbing my crayons and scribbling on my coloring book.

We also had brief exercise periods in a confined area outside the building. We often hit a volleyball around the group with the goal of keeping it from hitting the ground. A fellow patient would console me when I messed up and encourage me to start over. "It's all good," she would say.

She was a known troublemaker with the staff. Based on my own erratic behavior, I felt qualified to pass judgment. I remember thinking that she was destined for a much longer stay than me in the unit.

I became confused about what happened in the Quiet Room and tried to calculate when everything had happened. I was preoccupied with my fellow patients' comments and judgments.

Overly-sensitive to a peer's innocent remark, I complained to one of the staff. "Someone is starting stuff about me and I'm upset." After calming down, I returned to the lounge to watch television, and said, "I feel better now."

Per Amy's earlier advice, I was dressed in clothes, not pajamas. My most recent "voices" were three days ago, but I still believed that other patients knew my thoughts. I asked the staff to help me stop that from happening.

Specifically, one evening I experienced a bizarre incident when I wandered off. I was trying to read a magazine in private. There was an advertisement in it about taking a cruise to Alaska. Suddenly, I heard the other group members yell in unison from across the hall.

"Alaska!"

It totally freaked me out. I thought they were reading my mind. I was horrified, as I attempted to block my thoughts from them. I tried to stop myself from thinking, struggling in vain to cease imagining so much as a single thought . . . nothing!

This went on for about an hour. Every time I accidentally had a thought and they reacted with laughter in the other room, it only made me crazier. What if they really could read my innermost thoughts, and I was thinking something bad? What would become of me?

This reminded me of the night in the recording studio when I felt God had revealed the mental anguish in hell to me. We might be punished every time we had a single thought for the rest of eternity. Wow!

In case you're wondering why my fellow patients shouted "Alaska" in unison that night, I later found out they were watching *Jeopardy* and that happened to be one of the answers.

July 27 through July 29, 2003

I filed for disability while on the unit. It was later denied. I signed a consent form and letter to the Human Resources department at my job regarding when I would be able to return to work. My sister, Vicki, had been interfacing with them on my behalf throughout this ordeal.

I was still displaying signs of edginess in my room on the unit. I didn't feel safe with a recently admitted patient who scared me. I had to be coaxed to leave my room to watch television.

I still believed others could read my thoughts, but the paranoia was gradually starting to fade. I was social with a few patients, but I preferred to maintain a low profile. I continued to be leery of the newly admitted patient. My manic symptoms, especially my high rate of speed when conversing, continued to subside.

July 31 to August 1, 2003

As I neared the end of my hospitalization, I met with two of my sisters. I told them I felt about ninety percent up to par. I remained worried about returning to work and angry outbursts I might have, brought on by stress. I was determined to be more assertive toward coworkers in order to reduce anxiety.

The staff at the hospital suggested I continue to use a CPAP (Continuous Positive Airway Pressure) breathing device to treat my sleep apnea and loud snoring. I prepared for discharge the next day.

My Bipolar Disorder Psychiatric Diagnoses (During Four Hospital Stays) 1996/ 2000/ 2003/ 2003(b)

Psychiatric Diagnoses are categorized by the *Diagnostic and Statistical Manual of Mental Disorders, DSM-5*. This manual, published by the American Psychiatric Association, (2013) encompasses all mental health disorders for both children and adults.

The DSM-5 uses a multiaxial approach to diagnosing, since other factors in a person's life impact their mental health. It assesses the following five dimensions:

Axis I: Clinical Syndromes—This pertains to the actual patient diagnosis (e.g., bipolar disorder, depression, schizophrenia.)

Axis II: Developmental Disorders and Personality Disorders—The former includes autism, which is typically first evident in childhood. The latter are clinical syndromes that tend to have longer lasting symptoms and encompass the person's way of interacting with the world. They include paranoid, antisocial and borderline personality disorders.

Axis III: Physical Conditions—This includes conditions such as brain injury or HIV/AIDS that can result in symptoms of mental illness.

Axis IV: Severity of Psychosocial Stressors—Events in an individual's life, such as the death of a loved one or starting a new job can impact the disorders listed in Axis I and II.

Axis V: Highest Level of Functioning—This final axis measures the person's level of functioning both at the present time and the highest level within the previous year. Specifically, the Global Assessment of Functionality (GAF) is a numeric scale (1 through 100) used by mental health clinicians and physicians. It rates subjectively the social, occupational, and psychological functioning of adults. It measures how well or adaptively one is meeting various problems-in-living. The score is often given a range.

I found the DSM-5 model to be interesting when assessing my own diagnoses, which were assigned during my four hospitalizations. Several of them varied significantly, based on my admission and discharge summaries.

First Stay – September 27, 1996—October 3, 1996. Final diagnosis:

Axis I – Major depression, single episode, with psychotic features, and alcohol abuse.

Axis II – None.

Axis III – None.

Axis IV – Severe. Loss of job.

Axis V – Global Assessment of Functioning: 25 / 70.

Second Stay – March 9, 2000—March 22, 2000. Final diagnosis:

Axis I – Bipolar disorder, mixed with psychotic features.

Axis II – Deferred.

Axis III – None.

Axis IV – Moderate.

Axis V – Global Assessment of Functioning: 40.

<u>Third Stay</u> – July 3, 2003—July 14, 2003. **Initial** diagnosis:

Axis I – Bipolar disorder. Rule out paranoid schizophrenia.

Axis II – Diagnosis deferred.

Axis III – No diagnosis.

Axis IV – Psychosocial stressors: Unknown.

Axis V – Current Global Assessment of Functioning: 10.

<u>Third Stay</u> – July 3, 2003—July 14, 2003. **Final** diagnosis:

Axis I – Bipolar disorder. (Crossed out and marked as error.) Paranoid schizophrenia. [Note change from initial diagnosis.]

Axis II – No diagnosis.

Axis III – No diagnosis.

Axis IV – Moderate stress.

Axis V – Current Global Assessment of Functioning: 20.

<u>Fourth Stay</u> – July 14, 2003—August 1, 2003. Final diagnosis:

Axis I – Bipolar mania with psychosis.

Axis II – None.

Axis III – None.

Axis IV – Financial, occupational.

Axis V – Current Global Assessment of Functioning: 70. [Note improvement in my GAF rating from Third Stay to Fourth Stay only two weeks apart.]

Contemplating Electroconvulsive Therapy (ECT)

During my final hospital stay, I was initially uncertain as to whether I had undergone Electroconvulsive Therapy (ECT) in an effort to improve my recovery timeframe. This controversial procedure, which was also formerly known as shock treatment, can be defined as follows: "ECT is a biological procedure whereby a controlled amount of electrical charge is administered to the front part of the brain that helps certain kinds of psychiatric illness. Extensive research has shown ECT gives safe, effective, and rapid relief of symptoms for eighty to ninety percent of selected patients[44]."

My hospital records indicate that this procedure was recommended to me by my doctor, but that I rejected it. I opted instead for a change in medications, to include one that had only recently been approved by the Food and Drug Administration to treat paranoia. I had sunk so low into the depths of this bipolar episode that the medical staff was concerned my mental stability was tenuous.

There is a reference to me being administered Electrocardiogram (EKG) tests, which is probably where the confusion resides. This noninvasive, painless procedure records the electrical signals in your heart, and is used to detect heart problems.

I vaguely recall the placement of multiple sensors or electrodes being taped to my chest as part of some procedure. Marlene, also confirmed I was administered tests to monitor my condition.

In retrospect, just as I was beginning to slowly overcome my mental illness, I was noticing the early onset of Parkinsonian-type tremors. They initially manifested in my left pinky, moving to my remaining left fingers, hand, arm and leg. My head has since started to shake more frequently and now tilts slightly to one side. Although I would later be diagnosed with Parkinson's disease, there had been some initial doubt to the tremors' origin.

Several of my doctors have blamed this new medication as the source of these involuntary movements. However, after all these years, tremors have continued to occur predominantly on the left side of my body. Often in the early stages of Parkinson's, shaking is confined to one side, sometimes temporarily and other times permanently.

I continue to take the medication in question even today, since it is a key component in my bipolar treatment. If this is in fact a side effect of my pills, then the tremors are a necessary evil that I will struggle with for the rest of my life.

CLINICAL OVERVIEW (CHAPTER FOURTEEN)

*I*s Electroconvulsive Therapy (ECT) a safe alternative for treating bipolar disorder?

Electroconvulsive therapy (ECT) has existed since the early twentieth century. It's considered by some to be a very effective treatment for controlling and preventing bipolar episodes. However, therapy, medication, and lifestyle choices are commonly preferred solutions for addressing this illness on a long-term basis.

ECT has been known for decades to improve mood, although the misuse of this procedure in the past gave it a bad reputation. It is mainly used to treat the depressive phase of bipolar disorder, but can also be used during the manic phase. In some instances, it has been shown to be effective in preventing future episodes.

Although effective, ECT is usually reserved as a last resort or for special circumstances. It is often an option for people whose bipolar disorder has proven resistant to drug treatment or is causing severe episodes[45].

The immediate side effects of the procedure, which may last for about an hour, include: headaches, nausea, muscle aches and soreness, and disorientation and confusion. Patients may also develop memory loss. Memories formed closer to the time of ECT are at greater risk of being lost while those formed long before the program are at less risk of being forgotten. The ability to form new memories is also impaired after a course of ECT, but this ability usually makes a full recovery in the weeks and months following treatment.

During the actual procedure, the patient receives a minor anesthetic agent, which puts them to sleep for approximately five to ten minutes. A muscle relaxant is used to stop the muscles from moving during the seizure. Cardiac monitoring pads are placed on the patient's chest to check the heart throughout the procedure. Four electrodes are placed on the head. Two of the four monitor the brainwaves. The remaining two deliver a short, controlled set of electrical pulses for a few seconds. These pulses must produce a seizure to be effective[46].

It is important to note that, although ECT is considered safe by many in the medical profession, there is an alternative viewpoint. An organization known as the Citizens Commission on Human Rights (CCHR) reports that this treatment may have caused or contributed to multiple serious injuries or deaths. Specifically, this controversial procedure involves administering as much as 460 volts of electricity through the brain. It can result in cognitive impairment, prolonged seizures, dental trauma, pulmonary complications and death. In addition, one-third of ECT patients experience permanent memory loss and many suffer a steep drop in their IQ[47].

Based on these conflicting assessments, it is best to say that the jury is still out concerning whether ECT is a safe alternative for treating bipolar disorder.

FOURTH EPISODE

CHAPTER FIFTEEN FOURTH EPISODE – PART 1 GOODBYE TO STAFF

here were three nurses present when I left the hospital that final day in early August 2003. One of them said with a smile, "It was nice having you here . . . but we don't ever want to see you back here again."

Everyone chuckled. "That's right . . . you're not welcome back. Just take good care of yourself," another one chimed in.

One of them showed me a picture of a model in Cosmopolitan magazine. They told me she worked there at the hospital as a side job. I teased that I would like to have met her as one of my treating nurses. I began to blush at my own words, and we all shared another laugh. Then it was time to depart.

On the way home, Marlene and I picked up my meds. It had been a long, mind-bending nightmare of a trip away from home, spanning over one month. We arrived back at my apartment. I wasn't prepared to return to work, assuming I even still had a job after my long absence.

Marlene removed the thumbtack from my kitchen calendar and flipped the pages to August. "That's an experience in your life you won't ever want to look back on," she said.

I managed a smile: "You've got that right. Thanks for all your help."

"Well, I've gotta get going now. Are you gonna be okay?" She asked as she gave me a hug.

"Yeah, I'll be fine. I'll call you if I need you. Don't be a stranger." When she left, I flopped down exhausted on my living room couch. I noticed the room was now devoid of any signs of the Devil . . . no covens, no Buddha statues, no hairy trolls, no snakes, no gnomes, no Loch Ness Monster, no anything. I let out a sigh of relief as I shut my eyes and drifted into a light sleep, praying to God that my worst encounter with bipolar disorder was finally over. It was time to return to reality, whatever that was.

***

By the time I went back to work in September, I was still mentally and physically unsteady. I needed some additional rest at home. After finishing my extended stay as an inpatient in the psychiatric wards of the two hospitals, I was assigned intensive outpatient treatment at a third clinic for the month of August. Unfortunately, my records were destroyed and, for the most part, I can recall very little of this uneventful visit. By now, my management was pressuring me to return to the office or else face dismissal. My total hiatus from work had lasted more than two months. Because of the stigma associated with my bipolar illness, I stubbornly refused to reveal the nature of my prolonged absence. Instead, I blamed it on my difficulty to emotionally accept my father's death back in April. Almost five months had transpired since his passing and this story must have been getting more difficult to believe.

I returned on Monday, the day of our weekly staff meetings. Several colleagues passed insincere comments laughingly that increased my discomfort level.

"So, where've you been? We thought you had disappeared."

"Are you okay? You don't look right."

Others just gazed in my direction and chuckled, which was even worse. Several weeks later, I had to deliver a presentation to the salesforce in the conference room. I was in a comfortable setting and got to sit down throughout my talk. Even still, once I turned on the projector and began to speak, my voice cracked and I started to shake. I lost control of the audience. Everyone started to cackle. Even my best friend commented with pity, "Poor Steve." Obviously, their behavior was very unprofessional. I wished at that moment that I had admitted my bipolar condition upon my return to the office. Even though it was none of their business, maybe some of them would have been more sympathetic. I made it through the presentation, but it was a half-hearted effort on my part in the aftermath of the disruptiveness.

This incident wound up being one of the primary reasons I joined the Toastmasters public speaking group. A dozen years later, I won multiple public speaking awards in front of large audiences, but memories of that awful day in the conference room still linger.

On another occasion, I was embarrassed by my director during our weekly sales meeting. He insisted I stand at the white board in front of the room and take minutes of the meeting. Why couldn't I just remain in my seat and take notes on paper? Reluctantly, I went to the front of the room and began to scribble notes as best I could. My handwriting was becoming tinier and barely legible. Once again, everyone laughed at me. I was almost brought to tears.

My doctor prescribed valium to help me calm myself for these meetings. By now I was taking so many drugs, I was a walking zombie. I had hit the daily double: first I was walloped with a devastating mental condition, now I was hit with a still undiagnosed physical ailment. I wondered what would happen next.

Parkinson's disease increasing symptoms 2004

About a year later in 2004, I was driving when I suddenly noticed my left hand beginning to shake. I initially hoped it was a result of gripping the wheel too tightly, but deep inside I feared it was a possible initial manifestation of Parkinson's. Despite my concern, I stubbornly ignored the symptom for several months. What had started as a slight twitching in my left pinky was slowly spreading throughout my extremity.

I finally scheduled an appointment with a neurologist, who speculated the cause of my symptoms was one of my medications. Although it was new on the market, tremors were becoming a suspected side-effect.

When I followed up with my psychiatrist, he suggested that the shaking was a result of one of my other medications. The conflict of opinion was unsettling. Were either of the doctors correct? Over the subsequent years, my tremors gradually and sporadically increased. My right hand and arm would sometimes spasm, especially when I was writing or clenching an object or even in a resting position. My upper legs would also shake when confined in close quarters. I continued to refuse to seek further medical treatment. I was afraid of what I might discover.

The Year of the Cat 2004

In 2004, my family and friends convinced me to get a therapy pet to help me deal with my bipolar condition, even though I had never owned a pet in my life. I deliberated between a puppy and a kitten, but ultimately decided the latter would be less work.

It happened one Saturday, after searching multiple animal shelters —love at first sight. The smiling, attractive woman behind the counter of the shelter held a calico kitten in her hands, stroking it as it purred. Uncharacteristically, I got caught up in the moment and forgot that cute, playful kittens grow up to become shedding, troublesome cats. She placed the kitten back in its cage as she greeted me with a genuine grin. "Can I help you?"

Before I could respond, the front door swung open. In walked a heavyset, middle-aged woman and her young daughter, probably seven or eight years old. The girl gestured toward my kitten.

"Aw look, Mommy! That kitten is so cute. Can I pet him?" she asked the employee.

"It's a she," said the female worker as her face lit up. "And, of course you can pet her."

I felt myself slipping into a jealous rage. The mood stabilizers I had recently started taking weren't fully effective. My thoughts were much angrier than they should have been given the situation. I wondered almost audibly what that bratty kid thought she was doing, asking to play with my kitten.

I cleared my throat. "Excuse me, miss," I addressed the shop employee. "But I was here first."

The woman and her daughter's heads turned toward me. The kitten was clawing innocently at her cage door.

"You're not going to take that cute kitten away from my poor little daughter, are you, mister?" she asked in a confrontational tone.

I nodded, avoiding eye contact.

The woman swirled around and angrily confronted the employee behind the counter. "Are you going to let him do that?"

"I'm sorry, ma'am, but he was here first."

The woman glared at me as her daughter began to sob. "Well, I hope you're happy," she said. "You just broke my little girl's heart."

I mumbled an unapologetic, "I'm sorry," as she grabbed her young girl's hand and stormed out of the shop. I've never felt so rotten in my life and, unfortunately, my words would come back to haunt me. I am sorry I didn't walk away that day. My life over the next several years would be a nightmare with that frisky feline.

Company Plant Tour Circa 2005
Verbal Abuse at Work

Because of my perceived incompetency by most of my managers and fellow employees, I was switched back and forth between the sales department and product support at the manufacturing firm. I worked more than a year almost entirely engulfed in my severe third bipolar episode. Even though I could barely function each day, I managed to survive in the stressful environment for seven years and seven months. Between the rigors of having to meet my sales quota and ensure our product performed to our customers' satisfaction, the strain was unbearable. I avoided conflicts with my colleagues by distancing myself and hiding in my office. Some of them mistook this bipolar-induced shyness for rudeness and became angry.

I traveled quite a bit in my customer service technical position, even though I was not overly knowledgeable about the product. My business trips were throughout the country to our thirteen production plants. Most of these excursions occurred during my extended bipolar episode, placing me in several embarrassing and/or compromising positions over the years.

People are perceptive. From facial expressions and comments, I could tell they sensed something wasn't right with me. Some told me I didn't "add value" to the company. Others smirked when I didn't know the answer to a technical question. What annoyed me the most was that they thought I was dumb and as a result, showed me no respect.

I once traveled with two managers and a fellow sales representative. They knew I was a professed Evangelical Christian, not that I claimed to be perfect by any means. I was chastised at times by them and others for "not practicing what I preach."

One night these coworkers dragged me to a strip club. I told them I no longer drank. This was especially important since I was on multiple bipolar medications. Naturally, they ordered me a drink anyway. I set it down on the bar, feeling upset. The next thing I knew, one of them handed me a dollar as the dancer on stage shimmied in my direction. I reached up and somewhat clumsily gave it to her.

I turned to my coworkers and said, "C'mon, can we go now?"

But my night out on the town with the boys was just beginning. They paid one of the bouncers, who ushered me into the backroom for a lap dance. The girl was not my type, to say the least, with a pink, short-cropped haircut, and lip, tongue, and nose rings. They could have at least found me someone cute. I felt very uncomfortable for two reasons: my professed Christianity, and the fact that she was unattractive. There was a bouncer standing behind me in the curtained booth. At one point, he must have thought I was going to grab the girl because he yanked on my arm and scolded me, "Look, but don't touch." I thought to myself, there is a half-naked girl rocking back and forth on my lap, and Mr. Brawny is ordering me to look, but don't touch. Mercifully, my fun was soon over.

"Tip her, Steve! Tip her!" one of my colleagues pleaded as he stood in the doorway outside the backroom. He forced some dollar bills into my hand. But I turned and headed to the parking lot. They followed, annoyed.

Another Plant Tour Circa 2006

I visited another company facility for a major customer presentation and guided factory tour. The day before, I had traveled from the airport by car with one of our top sales reps, with the understanding that we would wake early the following morning for the show. It was critical that we assist with the setup before the dealers and distributors arrived. I had an early dinner at our hotel and was in bed by nine o'clock. The sales rep wound up drinking and entertaining his clients until two a.m. and slept in. I waited anxiously, pacing the lobby floor at seven a.m.

I called his room in a panic. "Roger, where are you? We're running behind!"

"Relax. You worry too much. We have plenty of time."

"I need a ride to the plant. You have the car. You're making me late!"

"Okay, okay. I'll be down in a minute . . . I'm just jumping in the shower."

Just jumping in the shower!

A half hour later, he finally stepped into the lobby and proceeded to order a leisurely breakfast. By now I was livid. When we finally left for the event, I didn't speak a word to him in the car. Sure enough, when we eventually arrived, the presentation was already underway.

My supervisor, who was overseeing the event, angrily pulled me to the side. "Where the hell were you? You were supposed to be here by eight!" she growled.

"I was riding with Roger . . . he made me late," I replied feebly.

"Bullshit. I'll deal with you later," she snarled, storming off.

I stood to the side throughout the entire presentation, dreading the pending consequences. Another manager glared at me. I could barely concentrate, and my thoughts became jumbled as I zoned out. My whole body was starting to shake, either from my Parkinson's, my bipolar disorder, or just plain ordinary stress.

When the agonizingly long presentation finally concluded, it was time for the plant tour and product demonstration portion of the event. A coworker displayed a small section of our plastic pipe to the dealers and distributors in the audience. I slipped into the back of the room inconspicuously after everyone else was seated and slumped in an empty chair with my head down, starting to nod off. Spotting me about to doze, my colleague tightly rolled up a piece of paper and loaded it into the pipe. He looked out at the crowd. "Watch this," He said. I felt a jolt slightly below my neck. Looking up, I realized what happened. He had shot a spitball across the room at me through the pipe, missing my face by inches. He garnered a few chuckles in the process. I guess this was my payback for being late.

It bears repeating at this juncture that, although I was now three years "officially" removed from my third and most mind-bending bipolar episode, I was still experiencing the ripple effect of my emotional earthquake. This seismic reading on the Richter scale had been the mental equivalent of a 9.0. According to the doctors in the psychiatric ward, they were almost unable to "bring me back" from the far reaches of my recent bipolar disorder assault.

In retrospect, I needed more recovery time before being capable of fully functioning in the corporate world. My nervous condition continued to worsen. My memory was shot. I was embarrassing myself with my apparent incompetency. If anyone belonged on disability, it was me, but my claim had already been long-since denied.

Music Career Revisited 2007

New Jersey remains the only state in the country without an official state song. In 1997, a contest was held to select a state song out of those submitted by two hundred contestants. My entry was titled "Greetings from New Jersey." Unfortunately, it didn't win, but neither did any of the other submissions.

Ten years later, I petitioned the New Jersey governor's office to initiate another contest to find a state song. Although I was unsuccessful, I approached the largest newspapers in my county to see if they would publicize my efforts. Two of them did so, one publishing a feature article with a front-page color photograph of me and my accompanying lyrics. This second New Jersey song of mine was titled "In the Garden State."

I received positive feedback from several assemblymen who saw the article and congratulated me on my latest attempt. I suppose my claim to fame is that my tune received airtime on a radio station in Trenton, the state capital. Although I have failed twice, I have not given up on my lifelong ambition to write the state song for New Jersey, my forever home.

The newspaper sent a reporter and camera crew to interview me at my townhouse in the early evening. My neighbors gathered on their front lawns to see the commotion. At least this time it was a happy commotion.

My Sister's Wedding Autumn 2007

Linda originally wanted me to be in her wedding party. I tried to convince her I was in no shape to do so since I was still in long-term recovery mode from my third and most volatile episode and hospitalization. I did reluctantly agree to escort our mother down the aisle, but my hands shook badly and I wouldn't be able to light the unity candles as she requested. I didn't want to embarrass myself and her in front of hundreds of people. Eventually, she understood, but the woman planner she had hired to arrange her wedding and reception did not.

I had the sole responsibility of driving my mother to the church. A bunch of us decided to follow each other since we didn't all have the directions. I tailed one of my nephews, but lost him shortly after a traffic light. My mother had advanced Alzheimer's disease, so she couldn't help. I remembered the name of the exit, but it headed both north and south. Naturally, I chose the wrong one more than once.

I traveled back and forth until I finally figured it out. I saw the church up ahead, but at this point, I had another problem. We were running about fifteen minutes late and holding up the entire ceremony. I plodded into the church with my mother, and practically had to drag her. Everyone had been wondering where the hell we were. The woman arranging the wedding was furious. She handed me a lighter and scowled. "Here, use this to light the unity candles when you get to the front."

As if she weren't angry enough, the expression on her face was frightening when I pulled away and responded, "I'd prefer if you have someone else light them instead."

She raged, "You're ruining everything." I moved forward sluggishly, with my mother grasping my arm, as I escorted her down the aisle. I remembered my earlier fear that the unity candles wouldn't light. I was right! When the wedding planner tried to light them, it took her, and eventually others, at least five minutes and many tries before the candles were lit.

The Cat from Hell

I had my cat for five years. Five long years. I knew she was going to be trouble when I couldn't even think of a suitable name for her. At first, I was certain we would be pals for life, so I named her Pally. After several misadventures over the years, I changed her name to Archie for reasons that should be evident based on my life story.

She proved to be anything but a stabilizing force in my bipolar episodic life. My biggest error in judgment was not having her declawed, a decision I made after being chastised by my niece, Kelly, that it would be inhumane. The cat refused to go to the vet for her shots. She scratched my furniture, including my recliner. She ran tight circles around my feet until I inadvertently stepped on her, whereupon she would howl like a wounded wolverine.

Eventually, I resorted to locking her in the basement, but she cried so loud she disturbed one of my neighbors, so I had to let her out. When I allowed her in my bedroom at night, she trampled my chest and clawed at my shirt. I locked her out of my bedroom, but she proceeded to jump up against the door handle until it popped open.

She ignored my mice and spit up fur balls everywhere. The last straw was when she began to pee on my pillows during the day when I was at work. I even resorted to putting old towels over the pillow cases, but when I arrived home, the towels were removed and I had to discard the ruined pillows.

Finally, I was able to lure her into my garage and lock her inside overnight. I called my friend Debbie and begged her to take the cat off my traumatized hands. Thankfully, she obliged. When Debbie arrived at my house, the cat willingly jumped into her waiting arms. Good riddance to my therapy pet that was supposed to comfort me. Debbie renamed the cat Buddy. And the story had a happy ending for all.

August 2008

In 2008, after having worked in the corporate world for more than twenty-five years, I decided to enter the human services field, mostly because I no longer wanted to work in a cutthroat industry.

My final stop in the business world ended after a long seven years. I was laid off when the company decided to relocate to the west coast to be closer to their overseas enterprise. Since the parent was worth over a billion dollars, I had worked for three of the largest corporations in the world: a major communications entity, a giant software firm, and now this huge manufacturer.

My honest-to-God intention going into my new "helping people" profession was that I wanted to interact with and assist the homeless and destitute members of society. This had always been a secret ambition of mine.

My first opportunity for this type of work was with a Catholic charitable organization. They offered me a job as a youth advisor in their Atlantic City facility. To be hired, I had to master the art of lying when I filled out several of the questions on the application form:

Have you ever been in jail/prison or convicted of a felony? If yes, please explain and give dates. My answer: No. (I didn't mention the four days I spent in jail because of a felony for allegedly assaulting a police officer when I was experiencing a bipolar episode. During the time period of the job application, I had been completing the expungement process.)

Do you take any medication on a regular basis?
No.
Are you currently under the care of a doctor?
No.
Have you ever had or do you currently have any of the following?
Suicidal ideation: No
Psychiatric Hospitalization: No
Depression: No

After repenting for these lies by reciting ten Hail Mary's and five Our Father's, I agreed to work as a volunteer for my first year, beginning in September 2008. As a repeat donor, I was familiar with the charity.

My corporate job had left me with a minimal severance package, which covered my living expenses in south Jersey for about four months. My residence was in a neighboring shore town island across the bridge from Atlantic City. When I accepted the volunteer position with the charitable organization, I no longer qualified for unemployment benefits, which were substantial. Prior to my most recent employment in the corporate world, I had twice made more than one hundred thousand dollars a year.

Over the next year, life in the shore house was somewhat of a soap opera with five roommates, four women and one guy. We all worked for the same charity. Another woman named Karen ran the volunteer program. She was very amiable, mature and professional. We seemed to get along.

My housemates were in their twenties. I was old enough to be their father. I didn't envision that to be an issue at first, since I had traveled the world several times with young people without a problem. This time was different. The only positive aspect of that first year was that my bipolar disorder was relatively calm. That would markedly change in year two. The bad news was my Parkinson's symptoms were becoming increasingly noticeable.

One night, the six of us were involved in an exercise to create heartfelt drawings for each other. We were asked to depict positive characteristics about our fellow housemates to promote unity within the group. My Parkinson's was escalating, but to maintain privacy, I still hadn't disclosed it to anyone. As I tried to write something complimentary about a fellow occupant named Helen, my hands shook uncontrollably. I scribbled a long line across the page and unintentionally ruined the drawing.

Once the exercise was completed, our instructions were to hang the colorful drawings on our bedroom doors. This would serve as a constant reminder of the importance of group unity. I couldn't help but notice Helen never hung hers up. My male housemate Jason privately told me she had referred to me as a *spaz,* because of this incident. I was disappointed in this hurtful remark. It was not a mature way to describe someone with a potential disorder.

In fairness to the rest of the volunteers, I didn't interact or mingle much with them the first six months we lived together. We often worked separate shifts at the shelter. Due to our age difference, I also quickly discovered that we had few mutual interests. And I had the insatiable hunger to hop on the bus into town every Sunday to watch the New Orleans Saints football games at a sports bar on the boardwalk.

I ran into some trouble with Karen, the woman who oversaw the volunteer program. I made an unwise decision to get close to one of the women in our house because I felt we had something in common. Beth Ann suffered from depression and often referred to her medication as *happy pills*. I had an error in judgment by overstepping my boundaries in our platonic relationship. Because I was twice her age, she viewed me as more of a father figure. Beth Ann and I purchased our meds from the same pharmacy on the small island. I was constantly afraid we would encounter each other there, and I wanted to maintain my privacy.

Although my medications were obviously being used to treat bipolar disorder, I wasn't certain who else in the group had guessed my situation. I was constantly experiencing mood swings, a warning sign that something was awry. Jason occasionally observed me popping my pills in our shared downstairs bathroom. He commented that I always seemed depressed. He was partially right.

2009/Early 2010

My Parkinson's symptoms continued to worsen. In hindsight, I'm not sure why I didn't address them sooner. I finally found a local doctor and began the process of treating my second malady with prescribed medications.

Around that time, a woman named Janice and two other female residents joined our group, replacing three of the original youth advisors who left our shore town. Janice was in her mid-fifties with a nasty disposition. She worked at the charitable organization in Atlantic City, as well.

I soon left the rank of volunteers and was now on salary, albeit minimal. I could afford a new place, so I set out on my own. My new work hours were strange in that my two days off were in the middle of the week. On one unseasonably cold and snowy day, my cellphone rang. It was Janice.

"Steve, I'm stranded at the bus station with no place to go. It's a long story, but can I please come stay at your house? It would just be for a couple days. I start a new job at the shelter next week. Please, come pick me up!"

"It's a blizzard outside. The bridge leaving the island might even be closed. How am I supposed to get to you and get us back safely? Besides, we've never even gotten along. You were nothing but rotten to me the whole year we lived together. I'm sorry, but the answer is no!"

There was a long pause on the other end of the line. For a moment, I thought she had hung up, but no such luck. "And you call yourself a Christian," she said.

I rolled my eyes and took a deep breath. "Okay. I can't believe I'm doing this, but I'm on my way. Hopefully, I'll make it." Fortunately, we returned to the house safely. She thanked me endlessly, like the hypocrite she was.

"But remember, this is only for a few days. Then it's time to go," I said.

"I understand, and thank you again so much."

Well . . . six months later, and she was still living in my house! Her supposed job offer had fallen through, and she couldn't find work. She had no other place to stay. Finally, Janice landed a job in the parking garage at one of the casinos and at least began to pay part of the rent.

She became the houseguest from hell who overstayed her welcome. If she wasn't hogging the bathroom, she was complaining to our upstairs neighbors for making too much noise. I tried calling the police to get her evicted. I hired a lawyer, who told me I'd have to pay to take her to court. Since I was renting the condominium, I had a clause stating I wasn't allowed to sublet. I was afraid I might get evicted if my landlady found out. The deeper I started to slip into my bipolar funk, the more I visualized Janice as the Devil.

***

One morning, I was steering my grocery cart around the corner of an aisle when I felt that familiar, indescribable feeling I wouldn't wish upon anyone. There were two stock clerks smiling widely, and I was certain they were laughing at me. Paranoia had set in.

I hurriedly finished my grocery shopping and raced into the parking lot. Before I even got in my car, I dialed my doctor's cellphone, leaving an urgent message. "Doctor, I feel like I'm losing it again. Please call me back!"

For some reason, I didn't care if anyone else was listening to my frantic plea for help. I just didn't want to fight my way through yet another bipolar episode.

My psychiatrist immediately returned my call. "What happened? Are you okay?"

"No, I'm not okay. Those Parkinson's pills must have clashed with my bipolar meds. I'm having an episode!"

"Okay, try to stay calm."

"I can't stay calm. I can't afford to have another episode."

"Where are you now?"

"I'm way down in south Jersey . . . far from your office." My voice rose.

"Which medication did your local Parkinson's doctor prescribe?"

"I don't know. He told me not to worry, that it was compatible with my bipolar meds. I guess he was wrong. I thought you said there wouldn't be trouble with his Parkinson's pills? You guys need to get new handheld devices to calculate these things correctly."

I ran my fingers through my hair and paced the parking lot.

"Can you call your Parkinson's doctor and have him give you your medical charts? There are always newer drugs for Parkinson's that may not cause a chemical imbalance like you're experiencing now. In the meantime, discontinue your Parkinson's meds immediately. I'll help hook you up with a specialist in north Jersey who is the best in the state. Are you okay to get by until tomorrow? Let's touch base again then. If need be, check yourself into a hospital down there."

Since I had detected the bipolar symptoms early, I thought I'd weathered the storm. Although it would be my mildest episode, it was not without incident.

Shortly thereafter, I met with the neurological specialist that my psychiatrist had referred me to in north Jersey. After extensive tests, it was agreed that I should switch to a newer medication. It wound up being a more effective alternative to my original Parkinson's meds. Unfortunately, my mental illness had received another blow. How much more could my battered brain absorb?

***

Although the Parkinson's medications were helpful, the entire left side of my body, arms and legs, still noticeably shook. I was also in the initial stages of another bout of bipolar that I had just experienced at the grocery store.

Only days had passed and already life had become unbearable, living in close quarters with someone I disliked. Before long, Janice was strutting around like she owned the joint. It was a small place, especially for two people.

When my fourth episode kicked in, I remember the song "Voices" by Chris Young was on the top of the country music charts. My irrepressible mania had me staying up late listening to the radio. I thought the lyrics in "Voices" were targeting me. Janice slept in my second bedroom on the other side of our shared wall. I would crank up the music just to interrupt her sleep. I was aware this wasn't Christian-like behavior, but it was the only means of retaining what little sanity I had left.

Another catchy tune played each night. The title escapes me, but I remember a verse about an Exxon gas station. I thought it was a strange lyric to have in a song, or maybe it was just a figment of my overly active imagination, since I was certain it was aimed at me personally. I thought the words were providing me with specific instructions.

Meanwhile, I was missing time at work. One night, I rummaged through the boxes in my basement, taking out a variety of ancient photographs, cards, and letters from former love interests, and remnants of collectibles. I was positive they harbored evil spirits. These thoughts brought back distant memories from a time my mother and brother insisted the items in my friend's overstuffed duffle bag were of the Devil.

I carried two black garbage bags containing this stuff and my daily trash out to my car and tossed them in the trunk. A mentally stable person would have simply thrown them in the dumpster up the block. Instead, my paranoia had returned in full force. My neighbor across the street had his bedroom light on. I was petrified that he was spying on me. So, I resorted to the only logical alternative. I hopped in my car and sped off down the road. My fifty-mile destination was Cape May! Yes, the voices from that song were instructing me to discard the bags in a dumpster across from an Exxon Station in Cape May.

With the hour approaching midnight, I obeyed the speed limit. I was deathly afraid of being pulled over and having to explain to a police officer where I was going at that hour. Not to mention two large garbage bags in my trunk. And why Cape May of all places?

Soon, I arrived at my destination, totally delusional. I spotted an Exxon station and I pulled into the lot. The problem was it was still open, and when the attendant saw my car approaching, he jumped up from his chair. I spun the car around and bolted before he could realize my intentions.

Not to worry—there was another Exxon station up the block. It was across from a busy nightclub blaring loud music. Many patrons were exiting the bar. Taxis waited outside. Horns were honking. There were people and cars passing by in every direction. There was also a huge dumpster, filled to the brim with white garbage bags. My two black bags would stand out on the white background like a Giant Panda.

It suddenly dawned on me. If someone were to open the bags, there was a vast number of items that would identify me, such as envelopes adorned with my home address. And if they decided to track me down, what plausible explanation could I possibly provide? What in blazes possessed me to drive my garbage all the way down the Garden State Parkway to dispose of it in Cape May? Bipolar disorder, that's what.

But now, it was too late. I had to move fast. I popped the trunk, catapulted from the car, and heaved the two black garbage bags on top of the pile of white ones. I lead-footed it down the road and made it home safely. Sometimes it could be an adrenaline rush to have bipolar disorder.

My Mouse Encounter

There's another goofy story that happened during my fourth and final episode. I sometimes had mice in my condominium down the shore. I was sleeping in my recliner one night, as I sometimes did.

I snore loudly and breathe through my mouth. My stomach was upset that night, as I was battling a virus. On top of everything else, I was experiencing a bad bipolar incident.

I awoke in the middle of the night and sprang out of my chair with a sudden urge to vomit, certain I felt something burrowing in my stomach. It must have crawled down my throat while I had my mouth open. It was a mouse!

It was approaching dawn as I dressed quickly and jumped in my car. I raced like a maniac down the road to the nearest hospital. I found my way to the emergency room and approached the window.

"Can I help you, sir?" The nurse asked, as if trying to guess my ailment since I had no telltale signs of one.

"Yes, miss. I swallowed a mouse!"

"You what?!"

"I'm pretty sure I swallowed a mouse!"

"Well, we'll have to set you up with an x-ray scan. Please be seated," She said with little emotion.

As I sat down and glanced around the room, there were people with broken bones, and bloodied bodies in obvious pain and discomfort. And here I was complaining about swallowing a mouse. They took a stomach x-ray and it showed nothing.

The doctor helped me maintain my pride by inquiring if it were possible I may have pooped the mouse out, which would explain why it was no longer present.

I had a much better explanation. I was crazy! I had become paranoid over the slightest thing. Now, I was worried I had swallowed a mouse! What had become of me?

CLINICAL OVERVIEW (CHAPTER FIFTEEN)

What is Parkinson's disease and its link to bipolar disorder?

In 1817 James Parkinson first described in his monograph, "Essay of the Shaking Palsy," the typical symptoms of Parkinsonism. The three cardinal symptoms are: tremor, bradykinesia (slowness), and rigidity (stiffness of limbs). If the initial presenting symptom is one of unexplained falls, it might be atypical Parkinsonism, as opposed to the most common form of Parkinson's disease (idiopathic). Parkinson's disease (PD) is a slowly progressive neurodegenerative disease that affects seven to ten million people worldwide. It is the second most prevalent disease of this nature. Alzheimer's dementia is first. The number of PD patients is expected to increase with the rising age of our population. It is slightly more common in men than in women.

Two out of the three motor symptoms make a diagnosis. A more recent nuclear medicine test, the DaTscan, can help confirm a PD diagnosis. The hallmark of PD is loss of dopamine, a neurotransmitter or chemical in the brain. Motor symptoms usually do not manifest themselves until dopamine levels are reduced by sixty to seventy percent. Symptoms are treated by replacing the dopamine with medication such as levodopa, which is the most effective.

POLAR EXTREMES

Though motor symptoms are what people usually associate with Parkinson's disease, many of the non-motor symptoms go unrecognized for years before a diagnosis is made. Although PD is a movement disorder, the diagnosis can be preceded or followed by psychiatric symptoms.

In some cases, bipolar disorder (BD) is linked with PD. Little is known of such comorbidities, and no treatment options have been recommended for such exceptional cases[48]. Theoretically, it is possible that major affective disorders may share some common pathophysiological mechanisms with PD. (Flemming, et al)[49]. In recent years, there has been increased reporting of cases of BD and PD occurring together[50].

The latest findings indicate a gene mutation that may create a risk for BD through a complex interaction of chemical signaling in the brain. This link between levels of neurotransmitters (nerve cells) can be associated with PD. Damage to vital organs (Mitochondria) that deliver energy to all cells has been found in brain imaging of bipolar patients. Roughly twenty percent of patients with this related disease also have BD[51]. Nerve cells were found to deteriorate in the brain area called Dorsal Raphe, which is a region also affected in Parkinson's, another condition that may have its roots in organ dysfunction.

CHAPTER SIXTEEN FOURTH EPISODE – PART 2 INCIDENT REPORT

O n the night of May 30, 2010 one of the shelter youths named Yvonne tested my authority as a resident advisor. She whipped the other youths into a frenzy and they started racing around the building, throwing pillows and making a mess. For the most part, they lived an unenviable, hard life in the "homeless" facility where I worked. However, the charitable foundation ensured that the youths were as comfortable as possible in their environment. The site was equipped with ten two-bedroom apartments, two big screen televisions, a full kitchen, a pool table, and other amenities.

Unfortunately, there were times like these when a situation could get quickly out of hand. Yvonne and the youths started throwing billiard balls at each other. They wouldn't stop, no matter how much I yelled. My whole body was trembling from the Parkinson's and the hazardous predicament that had escalated beyond my control.

"Look at Mr. Steve's arm shaking. He looks like he's starting to black!" shouted one of the male residents. This meant that I was becoming angrier.

I hurried into my supervisor's vacant office and locked the door. I called her for guidance. No sooner did I pick up the phone when the cue ball shattered the glass in her office door missing my head by inches. I thought, this isn't a bipolar hallucination. This is really happening!

My manager finally showed up at the facility to help restore order. She didn't offer me support and I was disciplined for this unfortunate incident. The glass was repaired the next day, and life returned to normal.

***

During the following day on May 31, multiple residents were sitting on the back porch listening to music. The mood was getting rowdy, and one of the back windows leading into the multi-purpose room had been opened. I suspected some of the youths had been drinking, but I was unable to confirm this. At one point, I heard a voice through the monitor intercom. "There's only one sip left in the bottle." As a result of all of the chaos from the night before, the youths had already lost all respect for me.

Immediately following this comment, another voice shushed the youth. Someone leaned against the back-porch camera, obstructing my vision. When I went to the rear of the building to investigate, I heard laughter coming from the kitchen. I entered the room and turned on the lights. I was shocked to discover two female youths attempting to engage in sexual activity.

Yvonne was sitting on the floor with her legs spread, dressed in a summer outfit, shorts and a T-shirt. Brianna was lying on her stomach with her mouth pressed against Yvonne's crotch, while trying to take off her clothing.

"I want to have sex with you!" Brianna said.

They both laughed as I tried in vain to verbally encourage them to separate. It was against agency policy for staff members to touch a youth. I tried turning the lights on, but that didn't help either. Yvonne reached up from her sitting position on the floor and turned them off. This happened several times. Eventually, I was finally able to convince them to stop. At one point, I heard Brianna declare, "I'm so fucked up!" I assumed this was from consuming too much alcohol. About five minutes later, I observed through the cameras the two women heading into Yvonne's apartment holding hands. The apartment door slammed, so I once again went to investigate. Before I reached the apartment, a resident friend of theirs named Raymond tried to verbally stop me.

"Mr. Steve, they're not in there."

"What are you talking about? I just saw them go in with my own eyes."

"Are you calling me a liar?" He persisted, following me closely.

By then my left arm had begun shaking violently between the effects of the Parkinson's disease and the renewed onset of bipolar disorder symptoms. I was flustered as to what to do next. I hadn't been trained to handle such a situation.

The apartment door was locked, so I opened it with my master key to find Yvonne laughing in a prone position on her bedroom floor. Hearing the commotion between Raymond and myself outside had apparently given Brianna the opportunity to hide. She had slipped into the shower stall.

I elected not to log this matter into the agency's computer, fearing the potential embarrassment it might cause the charitable organization should it ever be audited by an outside entity. But the situation was far from over.

On the following night, Brianna and Yvonne continued to tease me in the lounge area. On several occasions, they pretended to kiss each other while one of them lay down on the couch. At one point, Brianna lifted Yvonne's leg to try and get a reaction from me. When I glanced over to monitor the situation, she yelled, "I'm not stupid enough to try and have sex with her here in the lounge!"

Yvonne persisted in asking me why I had reported their lesbian activity to another staff member. This was the second time her primary resident staff member, one of my coworkers, had illegally repeated private staff-to-staff information.

On the following night of June 1st, Yvonne insisted I had attempted to get her in trouble. She added if I tried to get her suspended again, she would find out about it from her primary resident staff member. This comment alone made me reluctant to report future volatile incidents.

There was a saying among the residents, "Snitches get stitches and wind up in ditches." I was afraid my tires might get slashed.

Aftermath of Incident June 9, 2010

On Wednesday June 9th at our staff retreat held at a nearby college, I decided to tell the agency's management about the incident. There were four senior members of the organization present. I explained my account of what had occurred and my reasons for lacking the confidence to report the matter to my supervisors at the time.

During our brief meeting, we sat around a small cramped table. My Parkinson's symptoms flared up as they often did in close quarters. My legs kept rubbing together uncontrollably, causing them to spasm and bump against the managers' legs on either side. I became paranoid, fearing they would think I was nervous out of guilt. It was a very uncomfortable situation, so I finally just pulled my chair back from the table and extended my legs. It was only fitting I suppose. Here I was on a day when my bipolar condition was at bay, but my Parkinson's was acting up. I just couldn't win.

I restated my worries that an outside agency or the general public might discover that these incidents had taken place at our charitable organization, causing us embarrassment. I was notified that all investigations were conducted internally without the involvement of external auditing, so this wasn't a concern.

The following day I was suspended with pay for four working days, pending their investigation. On Wednesday June 16, 2010, I was called into a short meeting with my supervisor and manager. My employment was terminated despite never having been issued any warnings. The reason was my failure to properly report the incident in a timely manner. The two youths in question were never punished. It became apparent to me that the agency's management simply wanted me fired.

My corrective actions performance document contained virtually none of the required steps leading up to my termination. Specifically, I had received no informal dialogue, verbal warning, written warning, or extension of warning.

The document I received dictated the description of behavior or performance related issue as, "As a result of several written communications [untrue] and an admission by Steve [true] an investigation was initiated that determined that Steve failed to carry out numerous responsibilities of a Resident Advisor.

They are: stopping inappropriate client behavior on agency premises, demonstrating assertiveness and leadership, counseling clients appropriately in a timely fashion, documenting client incidents in a timely fashion and transitioning that information to necessary staff. The above incidents occurred after a number of supervision sessions with Steve that focused on the above responsibilities [untrue]. Steve has not demonstrated an ability to effectively carry out the responsibilities of the Resident Advisor."

I did eventually sign the document "admitting" my guilt because I was overwhelmed by the situation and by my illness. I lay sprawled on my bed, staring at the ceiling, alone with my thoughts. It had taken me several days to gather myself and respond to management's instructions to come to the office and sign the papers. My hand was shaking the whole time from the Parkinson's.

I had lost my job at the charitable organization, barely nine months after I started due to "poor job performance." Because I had essentially no income for calendar year 2009 as a volunteer, my unemployment benefits were zero. I also forfeited all company medical coverage because of my firing. I had been assigned crazy overnight shift hours at the shelter midway through my stay and, along with my overmedication albatross, I was often sluggish.

I hadn't been properly trained for my position, yet was expected to supervise fifteen to twenty rowdy youths on a daily basis. This task was undertaken mostly as a single advisor on the four o'clock to midnight shift. This included weekends and holidays when their unruly behavior was most difficult to manage.

In retrospect, I had devoted substantial amount of time and sacrificed a significant earning potential to volunteer my services to this agency. My initial seven-month period later developed into an approximate two-year stay that included my relocation to Atlantic City. Truly, my dream of helping those less fortunate and serving God wound up being a letdown. I encountered nothing but hypocrisy from within this organization. I left there disappointed that I had donated a single dollar of my earnings or a minute of my time to further their cause.

Winding Down in South Jersey
March 2011

After my days there drew to a close, my final job was at a small spiritual agency outside Atlantic City. I was in the heart of my fourth and last bipolar disorder setback. I was away from my doctor up north, and the long drive wasn't feasible. I didn't require hospitalization, but my meds were increased, making me feel incredibly drowsy.

My job title at this new agency was case manager, peer support specialist. It was a requirement of my position to have bipolar disorder. This was to help me relate to the members of my caseload as a fellow mentally ill consumer. It was a novel idea, since all of them suffered from a medical condition.

Craig was one of my clients who had severe bipolar disorder. With some help from management, I had secured him a nice second-floor bedroom in a sweet, elderly woman's house. There were immediate problems. My telephone would ring constantly from his landlady. For whatever reason, he was pouring bleach down the pipes, resulting in ongoing and sometimes permanent damage.

When I questioned him about it, he would look me straight in the eye and convincingly deny any guilt. "It wasn't me," he'd say. "It must have been somebody else."

Of course, there wasn't anybody else in the house who could have done it. Finally, after several similar incidents, my supervisor, Angela, suggested that maybe it was time for me to divulge to Craig that I also had bipolar disorder. This might form a bond, which would help to improve a bad situation. Unfortunately, this promising strategy wound up backfiring. I pulled him over to the side one day. "Craig," I said. "I'm not sure how to tell you this, so I'll just come right out and say it. I have bipolar disorder, too."

For a moment there was silence. I hoped for the best, but received the worst. He began laughing, but not in a happy way. He was ridiculing me "You mean you're bipolar too, and they sent you here to try and help me. You can't even help yourself." He turned his back and walked away.

When I told Angela what happened, she seemed surprised. "I'm sorry. That isn't how the peer specialist program is designed to work," she remarked compassionately.

"That's okay. I'm fine," I lied. "There's always a next time."

"I can understand why you'd be upset but, trust me, it happens to the best of us," she said encouragingly.

"I don't know," I half-whispered with my head down. "I'm just not sure I'm cut out for this type of work."

"Oh, c'mon, don't give up. It was one bad day. You'll bounce back tomorrow. You'll see."

I forced a smile, but the truth of the matter was that after three years in south Jersey, I had already decided to move back north. I would no longer live down the shore. My days working as a youth advisor and case manager in Atlantic City were over. I was in the process of completing my online Master's degree program in Human Services. I was homesick, especially with Christmas around the corner. Besides, I had been presented with an opportunity to work at a better paying job back home in north Jersey, so I accepted it.

It took over six months for me to get the bulk of my faculties back on track after leaving south Jersey. Prior to my departure, I had once gone to the bank to deposit my check with a blank stare on my face and my mouth hanging open. The tellers actually laughed at me. One of them bolted hysterically into the back room. And, this time, it wasn't paranoia on my part. It was really happening.

The same scene transpired at the post office. I was mailing a harmless package to a family member. The clerk witnessed that I appeared zombie-like, so she became suspicious of my intentions. She asked a straightforward question. "Does your package contain any explosives?"

I wasn't paying attention in my overly-medicated stupor, and I responded, "Yes, Ma'am."

She was understandably startled. "It *does* contain explosives?"

"Oh, no, no, no. I'm sorry. I misunderstood your question."

After what seemed like an eternity, I completed the transaction and safely made my way back to the car, forgetting the stamps I had intended to buy.

CLINICAL OVERVIEW (CHAPTER SIXTEEN)

W*hat are the health risks involved with misdiagnosis of bipolar disorder?*

Misdiagnosis of bipolar disorder (BD) is frequent in primary care practices. Early diagnosis of the disease is crucial for appropriate treatment and optimal outcomes, yet patients may go years without a proper conclusion. Furthermore, bipolar disease may begin as depression and develop into BD. Primary care physicians can watch for several red flags in patients with depressive episodes, such as poor functioning in social and work arenas, risky behaviors, and breaking the law. Other warning signs include a family history of BD, psychosis, or antidepressant-induced mania or hypomania. Correct and timely recognition of BD by primary care physicians can provide long-lasting benefits for the patient[52].

Bipolar disorder (BD) shares some symptoms with borderline personality disorder[53], a condition marked by impulsive behavior and social problems relating to other people. Because of this factor, people who have borderline personality disorder are often misdiagnosed as bipolar[54].

People misdiagnosed with BD may experience health setbacks as a result of the drugs used to treat it. Medications, including atypical

253

antipsychotics, can increase the risk for high cholesterol and diabetes. Some have also been linked to thyroid and kidney problems.

Up to twenty-one percent of people with BD may be mistakenly diagnosed with depression by their primary care doctors, according to a study published in the British Journal of Psychiatry[55] in 2011. A study published in Acta Psychiatrica Scandinavica[56] in February, 2013, found a gap of almost ten years, on average, between the participants' first onset of bipolar symptoms and their first treatment with mood-stabilizing medication.

"These findings aren't surprising," according to Jeremy Schwartz[57], a psychotherapist in Brooklyn, New York. "Bipolar disorder (BD) can be hard to diagnose,", he says, "because people often seek professional help only during their down periods and neglect to mention their up, or manic, periods . . . The manic side of BD isn't always bothersome to people," Schwartz says. "They have more energy, more motivation to do things. So the mental health professional doesn't always hear about it. As a consequence," Schwartz says, "those with BD are often misdiagnosed with depression and may be given inappropriate treatment."

"When bipolar disorder is missed, people can be put on medications that actually worsen the manic symptoms[58]," according to Schwartz. "So people end up waiting much longer to get the stability in their life that they're looking for[59]."

Should there be liabilities for doctors who prescribe wrong medications?

Psychiatric treatment can be a demanding, complex, and emotional experience for both doctor and patient. Because of the personal nature of the treatment, sometimes it is hard to tell when the doctor has committed malpractice.

Why is it important to differentiate between malpractice and the "medical standard of care," which absolves a physician from malpractice? Because in a successful malpractice case, the patient can recover money damages to compensate for injury, including emotional harm. Alternatives to a malpractice lawsuit include filing a human rights complaint, filing a complaint with the psychiatrist's employer, filing an ethics charge against the psychiatrist, writing negative online reviews for the psychiatrist, or speaking with the psychiatrist directly. However, these alternatives will not provide compensation to the patient for any harm inflicted.

To establish a malpractice lawsuit, a patient generally has to establish four elements:

- There was a doctor-patient relationship.
- The doctor breached the duty of medical standard of care (i.e., was negligent)
- The patient was injured (physically or mentally)
- There was a causal link between the negligence and the injury[60].

It is also important to note that a statute of limitations applies, which is the period after the alleged malpractice occurred and the time when the actual complaint was filed against the doctor.   This timeframe varies by state.

CHAPTER SEVENTEEN – EPILOGUE BACK UP NORTH WINTER 2012

I was still sluggish when I finally relocated back north in January 2012. All I wanted was to slumber like a hibernating bear. I drove to my brother's new house in the Poconos on weekends for Bible studies. However, no sooner would I arrive, when I would pass out on the carpeted floor. One time, his little daughter even chastised me by saying, "Why do you bother coming up here, Uncle Steve? All you ever do is sleep."

My final, milder bipolar episode was slowly fading. There were a few isolated incidents of paranoia that stubbornly remained throughout the next year. For example, I had entered a songwriters contest sponsored by a large record company. One of my songs, "On Bourbon Street," finished in first place in the Blues category. I was afraid they would steal my song and all its rights. I even hired an attorney to represent me in my lawsuit. The record label sent me a very polite letter stating that this had never been their intention, which made me feel foolish at first. Shortly thereafter, I discovered they had shut down their operations because of similar complaints concerning their tactics by other worried songwriters. My initial instincts had proved to be correct in the long run.

I was returning to my normal self, whatever that was. By now I had been struggling with bipolar disorder in excess of fifteen years. It felt good to be back home, living in a new rented condominium where I could finally achieve some semblance of sanity in my life.

The intermittent voices of Sonya, Cliff, and Priscilla were just a distant memory. Now the only voices I was hearing in my head when I awoke each day were those of Imus in the Morning, the New York-based syndicated talk show that played on my car radio. He and his crew entertained me during my seven to eight o'clock commute to the office. I was somehow able to relate to his stories of days gone by. I laughed at the crazy antics he had pulled while under the influence during his various episodes.

Whereas his episodes were self-induced by alcohol and drugs, mine were due to bipolar disorder. Nevertheless, it still drove home the point that we all share a common bond of attempting to cope with our inner demons. We somehow learn to survive in a mixed-up world whether we are celebrities or everyday folks.

I worked with moderate success as a grant writer for the next three and a half years at a school for special needs children. I secured a one hundred thousand dollar grant that allowed them to purchase an elevator. Overall, this experience wound up being a pleasant one. In mid-2015, I was laid off due to budgetary constraints. I enrolled for unemployment, and started an aggressive search for meaningful work.

My hopes were continually dashed as I chased opportunities in areas that reflected my strengths of the previous fifteen years. I was willing to accept positions in grant writing, fundraising, case management, customer service, or sales. I found nothing. In desperation, I even interviewed with a retail company in the grocery business. After glancing at my resume, one of their first questions was:

"Have you ever driven a forklift, Mr. West?"

I politely responded, "No, ma'am. I have not."

I was facing clear age discrimination. The fact that my left hand and arm noticeably tremored during interviews didn't help. I excelled at over-the-telephone interviews. When I sent a letter inquiring about a position, I was almost always able to reach the decision-maker through my persistent efforts, but still no job. I applied to over forty positions during an eighteen-month period with no viable offers. At sixty years old, there was no apparent reason to harbor hope.

I still sometimes ponder why I switched careers from the lucrative corporate world to the human services field. Deep down, I know the answer to that question. I wanted to devote the rest of my adult life assisting the less fortunate. Returning to school in 2011 to pursue my Master's degree in Human Services was a means of achieving this goal. The added stress this caused during my final episode was unbearable at times. However, I persevered and attained my diploma in 2013.

Finally, in 2016, I decided to accept a part-time position providing on-the-job-training for senior citizens seeking to join the workforce. The pay barely exceeded minimum wage, but I found it to be a rewarding experience. I was successful in placing adults in their fifties, sixties, and even seventies into gratifying occupations with hopes for career advancement. My involvement in this program covered two years. However, as of the writing of this book, my position has recently been terminated.

In early 2017, I became financially strapped as my life's savings dwindled near rock bottom. In desperation, I applied for permanent disability with the assistance of an attorney. He later reminded me that I had undertaken this process back in 2003 in the aftermath of my third and worst bipolar episode and been denied. However, with his legal advice, I gathered all available information pertaining to my history of mental illness to build a new case.

I discovered a brief journal I had maintained during that distant time period. I sifted through paperwork associated with my job terminations, and hospital discharge summaries. I collected information from sibling memories as well as my own. I successfully obtained all hospital records concerning my extended stays at three of the four facilities. It was at that time I conceived the idea to write this book.

But the clock was ticking as my savings account approached zero. In October 2017, my bank statement hovered around eight thousand dollars. I was nearing destitution. I calculated that I had enough money to survive another two months. And then what? I had no plan B. I prayed to God . . . often. Later that month, my prayers were answered when I received the call from Social Security telling me I'd been approved for permanent disability. My life carried on.

Later that year, I decided to join a writer's group in Morris County. I had recently self-published my first book, *"Tales of the Young West."* It contains my lifelong compilation of over three hundred original verses, short stories, lyrics, and comic strips encompassing more than forty-five years.

There are ten members in our group. Four of the others confessed to having relatives with bipolar disorder. If my math is correct, that's a fifty percent ratio, which makes me realize I am not alone.

***

By 2018, I had navigated my way through a rough stretch, first with bipolar disorder and later with Parkinson's disease. I'm hoping for a favorable outcome to my life story.

As this book neared completion, I was torn between retaining my bipolar secrecy of the past twenty-two years and opening the floodgates. My constant fear was that once I announced to the world that I have this stigmatic mental illness, there would be no second chance to put the genie back in the bottle. I would have "bared my soul to the crowd" in the words of Van Morrison from his epic single, "Why must I always explain?"

What if people laugh, ridicule, or avoid me? But I know I must stay focused on the bigger picture, the purpose for the remainder of my life. If my gamble reaps dividends, I plan to start a charitable foundation geared toward financially assisting society's mentally ill population, —many who exist behind closed doors.

I am a frequent visitor to the weekly local clandestine gatherings of these troubled people like myself. Because of their disability, many face financial ruin. I am determined to provide hope where there is only despair.

I also plan to use my hard-earned public speaking skills to help spread the word through educational talks. My ultimate goal is to start up a Christian ministry to further the cause.

In the meantime, I'm a survivor who will continue to write about the experiences on my emotional voyage, both the triumphs and the struggles. My faith in God will serve to guide me along the path to eternal salvation. I will start anew my life's journey with my four bipolar episodes, thankfully, far behind. I eagerly contemplate my travel plans. Someday soon, I will see the Grand Canyon. One day I will make it into heaven, but I will never, ever revisit the eerie, scary world of bipolar disorder.

Been there. Done that.

ACKNOWLEDGMENTS

Jennifer Walkup—Professional Copyeditor

Rob Palmer, Mira Peck, and Mark Vogel—Additional in-house copyediting

Carl Kline, Wendy Vandame, Nicole Yori, Tony Lusardi, Laura Oswald-Decker, and Nancy Heissenbuttel from The HighlandScribes writing group for their valuable input and feedback, including the Clinical Overviews

Charles Jijon—In-house copyediting, design layout/typesetting and formatting of the book/consulting

Mary Bawarski—Foreword

Chris Harrington—Cover design

Jacqueline Cristini, PA, MMSc, Director, Deep Brain Stimulation Program, JFK Neuroscience Institute, Edison, NJ—Parkinson's disease Clinical Overview

Dr. Lisa M. Steiner, Ph.D., LPC, LMHC, MBA, Director of Wellsprings Counseling Center, LLC, Fair Lawn, NJ—Research on Clinical Overviews 1-3

Tom West—Book title

REFERENCES

Aas, M., Henry, C., Andreassen, O., Bellivier, F., Melle, I., & Etain, B. (2016). The Role of Childhood Trauma in Bipolar Disorders. *International Journal of Bipolar Disorders, 4*(1), 1-10.

American Academy of Child and Adolescent Psychiatry. (2015). *What causes pediatric bipolar disorder?* Retrieved May 22, 2017, from www.aacap.org: https://www.aacap.org/AACAP/Families_and_Youth/Resource_Centers/Bipolar_Disorder_Resource_Center/FAQ.aspx#bipolarfaq1

American Foundation of Suicide Prevention. (2016). *Risk Factors and Warning Signs*. Retrieved June 17, 2017, from American Foundation of Suicide Prevention: https://afsp.org/about-suicide/risk-factors-and-warning-signs/

American Foundation of Suicide Prevention. (2017). *Suicide Statistics*. Retrieved 12 22, 2018, from AFSP: https://afsp.org/about-suicide/suicide-statistics/

American Psychatric Association. (2013). In *Diagnostic and Statistical Manual of Menter Disorders: DSM-5* (p. 123). Washington, DC: American Psychiatric Association.

Andreasen, N. C. (2008, June). The relationship between creativity and mood disorders. *Dialogues in clinical neuroscience, 10*(2), 251-255. Retrieved from https://www.ncbi.nlm.nih.gov/pmc/articles/PMC3181877/

Baldessarini, R., Pompili, M., & Tondo, L. (2006). Suicide in Bipolar Disorder: Risks and Management. *CNS Spectr, 11*(6), 465-471.

Bipolar Lives. (n.d.). *Bipolar disorder and creativity*. Retrieved December 29, 2018, from bipolor-lives.com: www.bipolar-lives.com/bipolar-disorder-and-creativity.html

BipolarLives.com. (n.d.). *Bipolar Disorder and Creativity*. Retrieved 12 18, 2018, from https://www.bipolar-lives.com/bipolar-disorder-and-creativity.html

Carrier Clinic. (n.d.). *Electroconvulsive Therapy (ECT)*. Retrieved from CarrierClinic.org: https://carrierclinic.org/programs/electro-convulsive-therapy/

Citizens Commission on Human Rights. (n.d.). *ECT Device Producer Flouts FDA Regulations*. Retrieved from www.cchr.org: http://www.cchr.org/newsletter/issue12/ect-device-producer-flouts-fda-regulations.html

Collingwood, J. (n.d.). *The Link Between Bipolar Disorder and Creativity*. Retrieved December 29, 2018, from PsychCentral: https://psychcentral.com/lib/the-link-between-bipolar-disorder-and-creativity/

Culpepper, L. (2014). Misdiagnosis of Bipolar Depression in Primary Care Practices. *The Journal of Clinical Psychiatry, 75*(3). Retrieved from http://www.psychiatrist.com/JCP/article/Pages/2014/v75n03/v75n03e05.aspx

Depression and Bipolar Support Alliance. (n.d.). *Homepage*. Retrieved December 29, 2018, from DBSA: https://secure2.convio.net/dabsa/site/SPageServer/PageServer?pagename=home

Diep, F. (2017, Sep 11). *What Happens When You Stop Taking Psychiatric Medications*. Retrieved from Pacific Standard: https://psmag.com/news/what-happens-when-you-stop-taking-psychiatric-medications

Drancourt, N., Etain, B., Lajnef, M., Henry, C., Raust, A., Cochet, B., . . . Bellivier, F. (2013, Feb). Duration of untreated bipolar disorder: missed opportunities on the long road to optimal treatment. *Acta Psychiatrica Scandinavica, 127*(2), 136-44. Retrieved from https://www.ncbi.nlm.nih.gov/pubmed/22901015

Duntley, J. D. (2005). *Homicidal Ideation.* University of Texas at Austin. Retrieved from University of Texas Libraries: http://legacy.lib.utexas.edu/etd/d/2005/duntleyj48072/duntleyj48072.pdf

Engmann, B. (2011, October 19). Case Report: Bipolar Affective Disorder and Parkinson's Disease. (A. M. Sharma, Ed.) *Case Reports in Medicine, 2011.* doi:http://dx.doi.org/10.1155/2011/154165

Flemming, M. N. (2012, January). Parkinson's disease and affective disorder: The temporal relationship. *Open Journal of Psychiatry, 02*(02), 96-109. doi:10.4236/ojpsych.2012.22014

Foundations Recovery Network. (n.d.). *Bipolar Disorder and Addiction.* Retrieved December 26, 2018, from DualDiagnosis.org: www.dualdiagnosis.org/bipolar-disorder-and-addiction/

Ghouse, A. A., Sanches, M., Zunta-Soares, G., Swann, A. C., & Soares, J. C. (2013, September 23). Overdiagnosis of Bipolar Disorder: A Critical Analysis of the Literature. (W. M. Bahk, C. M. Beasley, & H. Hori, Eds.) *The Scientific World Journal, 2013.* doi:http://dx.doi.org/10.1155/2013/297087

Howard, G. (2017, April 25). *3 Simple Ways to Explain Bipolar Disorder to Others.* Retrieved from bphope.com: www.bphope.com/blog/3-simple-ways-to-explain-bipolar-disorder-to-others/

Johns Hopkins Medicine. (n.d.). *Brain Stimulation*. Retrieved from www.hopkinsmedicine.org: https://www.hopkinsmedicine.org/psychiatry/specialty_areas/brain_stimulation/ect/faq_ect.html

Johnson, R. L. (2015, June 24). *When to Sue Your Psychiatrist for Malpractice*. Retrieved from Psychology Today: https://www.psychologytoday.com/us/blog/so-sue-me/201506/when-sue-your-psychiatrist-malpractice

Koenig, H. (2009, May). Research on religion, spirituality and mental health: a review. *Canadian Journal of Psychiatry, 54*(5), 283-291. Retrieved from PubMed.gove: https://www.ncbi.nlm.nih.gov/pubmed/19497160

Lawler, M. (n.d.). *6 Signs You or Someone You Know Has Borderline Personality Disorder*. Retrieved Jan 20, 2019, from EverydayHealth.com: https://www.everydayhealth.com/bpd/guide/symptoms/

Livingston, J. D. (2016, August 1). Contact Between Police and People With Mental Disorders: A Review of Rates. *Psychiatric Services, 67*(8), 850-857. Retrieved from https://ps.psychiatryonline.org/doi/full/10.1176/appi.ps.201500312

Mann, D. (n.d.). *The Dangerous Side of Mania*. Retrieved from EverydayHealth.com: https://www.everydayhealth.com/news/dangerous-side-mania/

Mayo Clinic. (n.d.). *Electroconvulsive Therapy (ECT)*. Retrieved from MayoClinic.org: https://www.mayoclinic.org/tests-procedures/electroconvulsive-therapy/about/pac-20393894

McCormick, U., Murray, B., & McNew, B. (2015, Sep). Diagnosis and treatment of patients with bipolar disorder: A review for advanced practice nurses. *Journal of the American Association of Nurse Practitioners, 27*(9), 530-542. Retrieved from https://www.ncbi.nlm.nih.gov/pmc/articles/PMC5034840/

McGovern, M., Xie, H., Segal, S., Siembab, L., & Drake, R. (2006, October). Addiction treatment services and co-occurring disorders: Prevalence estimates, treatment practices, and barriers. *Journal of Substance Abuse Treatment, 31*(3), 267-275. doi:https://doi.org/10.1016/j.jsat.2006.05.003

Melancholia, J. (2016, March 24). *Suicide: Bipolar Depression's Last Trick.* Retrieved from www.bphope.com: https://www.bphope.com/blog/suicide-bipolar-depressions-last-trick/

National Alliance on Mental Illness. (2017). *Bipolar Disorder.* Retrieved 12 22, 2018, from NAMI: https://www.nami.org/Learn-More/Mental-Health-Conditions/Bipolar-Disorder/Overview

National Alliance on Mental Illness. (n.d.). *About NAMI.* Retrieved December 30, 2018, from nami.org: https://www.nami.org/About-Nami

National Alliance on Mental Illness. (n.d.). *Bipolar Disorder.* Retrieved from nami.org: https://www.nami.org/learn-more/mental-health-conditions/bipolar-disorder

National Alliance on Mental Illness. (n.d.). *Find Support.* Retrieved December 29, 2018, from nami.org: https://www.nami.org/Find-Support

National Alliance on Mental Illness. (n.d.). *Mental Health Medications.* Retrieved from www.nami.org: https://www.nami.org/Learn-More/Treatment/Mental-Health-Medications

National Alliance on Mental Illness. (n.d.). *Schizoaffective Disorder.* Retrieved from nami.org: www.nami.org/learn-more/mental-health-conditions/schizoaffective-disorder

National Institute of Mental Health. (2015). *Bipolar Disorder in Children and Teens*. Retrieved May 22, 2017, from nimh.nih.gov: https://www.nimh.nih.gov/health/publications/bipolar-disorder-in-children-and-teens/index.shtml

Novaretti, T. M., Novaretti, N., & Tumas, V. (2016, Oct-Dec). Bipolar disorder, a precursor of Parkinson's disease? *Dementia & Neropsychologia, 10*(4), 361-364. doi:https://dx.doi.org/10.1590%2Fs1980-5764-2016dn1004018

Owen, R., Gooding, P., Dempsey, R., & Jones, S. (2017, July). The Reciprocal Relationship between Bipolar Disorder and Social Interaction: A Qualitative Investigation. *Clinical Psychology and Psychotherapy, 24*(4), 911-918. Retrieved from https://www.nami.org/Find-Support

Rush University Medical Center. (2010, Feb 24). *Belief in a caring god improves response to medical treatment for depression, study finds*. Retrieved from ScienceDaily: https://www.sciencedaily.com/releases/2010/02/100223132021.htm

Sample, I. (2015, Jun 8). *New study claims to find genetic link between creativity and mental illness*. Retrieved from TheGuardian.com: https://www.theguardian.com/science/2015/jun/08/new-study-claims-to-find-genetic-link-between-creativity-and-mental-illness

Schwartz, J. (n.d.). *Welcome*. Retrieved from ParkSlopeTherapy.net: https://www.parkslopetherapy.net/p/welcome.html

ScienceDaily. (2018, June 11). *Mutation links bipolar disorder to mitochondrial disease*. Retrieved from www.sciencedaily.org: https://www.sciencedaily.com/releases/2018/06/180611133414.htm

Scott, J. A. (n.d.). *Why Bipolar Disorder Is Often Wrongly Diagnosed.* (A. Young, Editor) Retrieved 05 15, 2015, from www.everydayhealth.com: https://www.everydayhealth.com/news/why-bipolar-disorder-is-often-misdiagnosed/

Sher, L., Rice, T., & Health, W. F. (2015). Prevention of homicidal behaviour in men with psychiatric disorders. *The World Journal of Biological Psychiatry, 16*(4), 212-229. Retrieved from https://www.google.com/url?sa=t&source=web&rct=j&url=http://www.wfsbp.org/fileadmin/user_upload/Treatment_Guidelines/2015_Sher_et_al.pdf&ved=2ahUKEwiY5s-5r8XbAhXCk1kKHchtCYcQFjAIegQIBRAB&usg=AOvVaw3qs5xU7UFPJdFItsqHlxtz

Smith, D. J., Griffiths, E., Kelly, M., & Hood, K. (2011, July). Unrecognized bipolar disorder in primary care patients with depression. *The British Journal of Psychiatry, 199*(1), 49-56. doi:https://doi.org/10.1192/bjp.bp.110.083840

Sonne, S. C., & Brady, K. T. (2002). *Bipolar Disorder and Alcoholism.* Retrieved Dec 26, 2018, from National Institute on Alcohol Abuse and Alcoholism: https://pubs.niaaa.nih.gov/publications/arh26-2/103-108.htm

Starzer, M. S., Nordentoft, M., & Hjorthoj, C. (2018, Apr). Rates and Predictors of Conversion to Schizophrenia or Bipolar Disorder Following Substance-Induced Psychosis. *The American Journal of Psychiatry, 175*(4), 343-350. doi:https://doi.org/10.1176/appi.ajp.2017.17020223

Szabo, L. (2015, December 10). *People with mental illness 16 times more likely to be killed by police.* Retrieved from USA Today: www.usatoday.com/story/news/2015/12/10/people-mental-illness-16-times-more-likely-killed-police/77059710/

Thienhaus, O. J., & Piasecki, M. (1998, September). Assessment of Psychiatric Patients' Risk of Violence Toward Others. *Psychiatric Services, 49*(9), 1129-1147. doi:https://doi.org/10.1176/ps.49.9.1129

Tondo, L., Pompili, M., Forte, A., & Baldessarini, R. J. (2016). Suicide Attempts in Bipolar Disorders: Comprehensive Review of 101 Reports. *Acta Psychiatrica Scandinavia, 133*, 174-186.

Tracy, N. (n.d.). *Effects of Bipolar Disorder on Family and Friends*. Retrieved December 30, 2018, from HealthyPlace.com: healthyplace.com/bipolar-disorder/bipolar-support/effects-of-bipolar-disorder-on-family-and-friends/

Tracy, N. (n.d.). *Living with Bipolar and Living with Someone Who is Bipolar*. Retrieved December 30, 2018, from HealthyPlace.com: https://www.healthyplace.com/bipolar-disorder/bipolar-support/living-with-bipolar-and-living-with-someone-who-is-bipolar

University of Florida Health. (n.d.). *Bipolar Disorder*. Retrieved Dec 26, 2018, from ufhealth.org: m.ufhealth.org/bipolar-disorder

END NOTES

[1] (American Psychatric Association, 2013)

[2] (American Psychatric Association, 2013, p. 124)

[3] (National Alliance on Mental Illness, 2017)

[4] (American Psychatric Association, 2013)

[5] (American Foundation of Suicide Prevention, 2017)

[6] (Baldessarini, Pompili, & Tondo, 2006)

[7] (Tondo, Pompili, Forte, & Baldessarini, 2016)

[8] (American Foundation of Suicide Prevention, 2016)

[9] (American Psychatric Association, 2013)

[10] (American Academy of Child and Adolescent Psychiatry, 2015)

[11] (Aas, et al., 2016)

[12] (National Institute of Mental Health, 2015)

[13] (Sonne & Brady, 2002)

[14] (McGovern, Xie, Segal, Siembab, & Drake, 2006)

[15] (American Psychatric Association, 2013)

[16] (Starzer, Nordentoft, & Hjorthoj, 2018)

[17] (Foundations Recovery Network, n.d.)

[18] (McCormick, Murray, & McNew, 2015)

[19] (University of Florida Health, n.d.)

[20] (Diep, 2017)

[21] (Rush University Medical Center, 2010)

[22] (Koenig, 2009)

[23] (Duntley, 2005, pp. 51-55)

[24] (Thienhaus & Piasecki, 1998)

[25] (Sher, Rice, & Health, 2015)

[26] (Sample, 2015)

[27] (Andreasen, 2008)

[28] (Bipolar Lives, n.d.)

[29] (Collingwood, n.d.)

[30] (Howard, 2017)

[31] (Melancholia, 2016)

[32] (Depression and Bipolar Support Alliance, n.d.)

[33] (National Alliance on Mental Illness, n.d.)

[34] (Owen, Gooding, Dempsey, & Jones, 2017)

[35] (Tracy, Effects of Bipolar Disorder on Family and Friends, n.d.)

[36] (Tracy, Living with Bipolar and Living with Someone Who is Bipolar, n.d.)

[37] (National Alliance on Mental Illness, n.d.)

[38] (Depression and Bipolar Support Alliance, n.d.)

[39] (Szabo, 2015)

[40] (Livingston, 2016)

[41] (National Alliance on Mental Illness, n.d.)

[42] (National Alliance on Mental Illness, n.d.)

[43] (National Alliance on Mental Illness, n.d.)

[44] (Carrier Clinic, n.d.)

[45] (Mayo Clinic, n.d.)

[46] (Johns Hopkins Medicine, n.d.)

[47] (Citizens Commission on Human Rights, n.d.)

[48] (Engmann, 2011)

[49] (Flemming, 2012)

[50] (Novaretti, Novaretti, & Tumas, 2016)

[51] (ScienceDaily, 2018)

[52] (Culpepper, 2014)

[53] (Lawler, n.d.)

[54] (Ghouse, Sanches, Zunta-Soares, Swann, & Soares, 2013)

[55] (Smith, Griffiths, Kelly, & Hood, 2011)

[56] (Drancourt, et al., 2013)

[57] (Schwartz, n.d.)

58 (Mann, n.d.)
59 (Scott, n.d.)
60 (Johnson, 2015)

53179880R00164

Made in the USA
Columbia, SC
15 March 2019